Type II Diabetes:
Your Healthy Living Guide

TYPE II DIABETES: YOUR HEALTHY LIVING GUIDE

American Diabetes Association

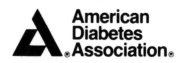

Printed in the United States of America

American Diabetes Association
1660 Duke Street
Alexandria, Virginia 22314

Library of Congress Cataloging-in-Publication Data

Type II diabetes.

    Includes index.
    1. Non-insulin-dependent diabetes--Popular works.
I. American Diabetes Association. {DNLM: 1. Diabetes
Mellitus, Non-Insulin-Dependent--popular works.
WK 810 T991}
RC660.4T97 1992   616.4'62   92-17906
ISBN 0-945448-27-9 (pbk.)

The mission of the American
Diabetes Association is
to prevent and cure diabetes
and to improve the lives
of all people affected by diabetes.

TABLE OF CONTENTS

ACKNOWLEDGMENTS

Just as type II diabetes is complicated, so is writing about it. The information in *Type II Diabetes: Your Healthy Living Guide* first appeared in the American Diabetes Association publications *Diabetes Forecast, Diabetes Care, Diabetes Spectrum,* and *Therapy of Diabetes Mellitus and Related Disorders.* Managing Editor Christine B. Welch, along with writers Amanda Patton and Sharon Block, adapted this information into this sourcebook on type II diabetes. Sue Thom, RD, LD, CDE (Saint Vincent Charity Hospital, Cleveland, Ohio) and Nancy Cooper, RD (International Diabetes Center, Minneapolis, Minnesota) provided much information on making healthy food choices.

The detailed and thoughtful comments of the reviewers kept this book relevant to the real concerns of people with type II diabetes. We thank all of these reviewers, professionals who spend their lives caring for individuals with type II diabetes:

Saul Genuth, MD
The Mt. Sinai Medical Center
Cleveland, Ohio

Steven V. Edelman, MD
Veteran Affairs Medical
    Center
San Diego, California

Dorothea F. Sims
South Burlington, Vermont

Ethan A.H. Sims, MD
College of Medicine,
    University of Vermont
Burlington, Vermont

Laura Renfrow, RN, MA,
    CDE
Diabetes Center of the
    Medical Center of Central
    Massachusetts
Worchester, Massachusetts

Jaime A. Davidson, MD,
    FACP
Endocrine & Diabetes
    Associates of Texas
Dallas, Texas

Joan Fitzgerald, RN, MSN,
    FNP, CDE
Veterans Affairs Medical
    Center
San Diego, California

Lorraine C. Schafer, PhD
Mayo Clinic
Rochester, Minnesota

John Colwell, MD, PhD
Medical University of South
    Carolina
Charleston, South Carolina

Davida F. Kruger, MSN,
  RN, CDE
Henry Ford Hospital
Detroit, Michigan

Aubrey E. Boyd III, MD
Tufts New England Medical
  Center
Boston, Massachusetts

Many people at the American Diabetes Association National Center contributed to this book. Thanks go to Peter Banks, Editorial Director; Kim Fawcett, Production Manager; Phyllis Barrier, MS, RD, CDE, Director of Council Affairs; Susan H. Lau, Publisher; and Richard Kahn, PhD, Chief Scientific and Medical Officer.

We are grateful to Alan K. Richards and colleagues at the Health Insurance Association of America (Washington, DC) for verifying information about health insurance.

Book design is by RCW Communication Design, Inc. (Falls Church, Virginia). Illustrations are by Gary Davis (Wakefield, Massachusetts).

INTRODUCTION

ABOUT THIS BOOK

This book is a result of the American Diabetes Association's mission: to prevent and cure diabetes and to improve the lives of all people affected by diabetes.

The American Diabetes Association believes in the highest standards of health care for people with diabetes. *Type II Diabetes: Your Healthy Living Guide* takes these standards of care and shows you how to apply them to obtain the best possible care for type II diabetes. Because we are committed to the best possible care, our standards are high.

We believe that everyone with diabetes should have access to a health-care team: a primary care physician with interest and experience in diabetes care (preferably an endocrinologist), a dietitian, an eye-care specialist, a diabetes educator, a mental health professional, a podiatrist, and an exercise specialist. This is an ideal in diabetes care.

You may find that your community does not have the resources to provide you with the services or professionals we would like you to have. Like most Americans, you may be financially limited in the kinds of health care you can seek. However, we want you to know what to aim for in your diabetes care.

Even if you see just one medical professional for all your diabetes care, you still need to receive proper foot care and eye care, an exercise prescription that is safe for you, a comprehensive meal plan, and medications. You need to be educated about diabetes and diabetes care. You should not be on your own.

This book contains a list of resources you may find helpful in achieving good diabetes care. The list contains the names of some publications we feel are extremely valuable and associations that can give you assistance in overcoming your particular hurdles. If you get "stuck" for any reason, your first call should be to the American Diabetes Association, listed in the white pages of your phone book.

The people featured in this book are real. Their thoughts and stories have been published in *Diabetes Forecast*, the members' magazine of the American Diabetes Association. Seeing diabetes through their eyes may help remind you that you are not alone in your struggle to live a healthy life with diabetes.

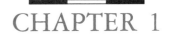

CHAPTER 1

Type II Diabetes

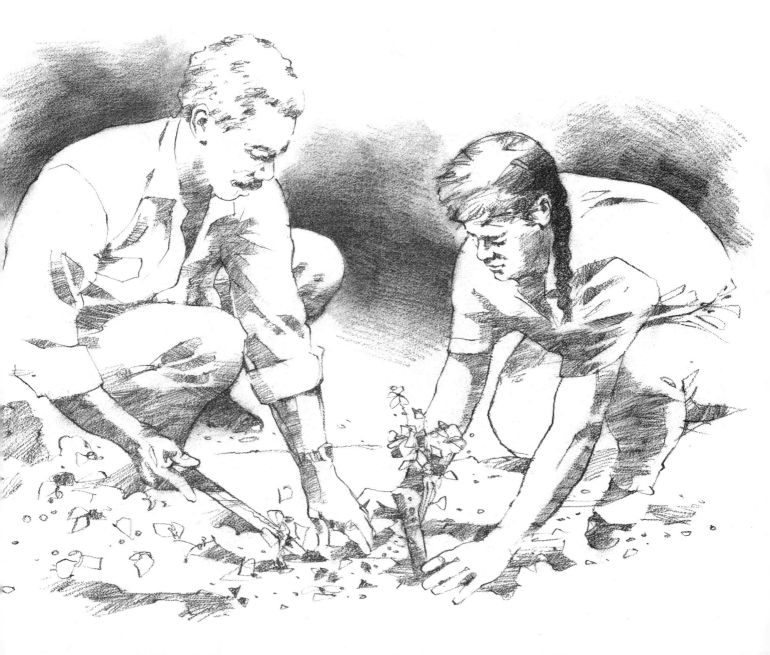

How did you learn that you have type II diabetes? Did the classic symptoms of frequent urination, unusual thirst, excessive fatigue, blurry vision, weight loss, and persistent infections get you to the doctor? Or were you surprised to find you had diabetes when you were visiting your doctor about your shortness of breath or pain in your legs or during a routine checkup? Maybe your physician had warned you some time back to lose weight, that you could develop diabetes?

More people have diabetes than ever before. In, fact one in every 20 people has the disease. In the United States, type II diabetes, also known as non-insulin-dependent diabetes mellitus, accounts for more than 95 percent of all cases of diabetes — or over 13 million Americans. Half of these people don't even know they have diabetes. So, you're not alone!

But, why you?

Are you overweight? Three of four people diagnosed with type II diabetes are or were obese. Obesity means weighing 20 percent more than your healthy body weight. Leading a sedentary, "couch potato" life contributes to obesity. Type II diabetes can occur in normal-weight people, too — people who have small muscles and extra body fat. **Where** you're fat is also important. Carrying excess fat above the hips is related to increased risk of developing type II diabetes.

Was diabetes diagnosed in your parents or grandparents? Your ancestors may have died of diabetes without even knowing it — the accompanying diseases of diabetes, called complications, such as heart disease and kidney failure, could have been listed as the cause of death. Type II diabetes "runs" in families. Many people with type II diabetes have parents or siblings who also have type II diabetes. Almost certainly, there are one or more genes that make individuals susceptible to developing type II diabetes. Although the "type II diabetes genes" haven't been discovered yet, your family background, whether through inherited traits or learned habits, plays a big role.

Are you over 30 years old? The risk of type II diabetes becomes larger as age increases. Half of the people with diabetes are over 55.

Are you American Indian, Black, or Hispanic? As many ethnic groups were exposed to the common lifestyle of the U.S.

in the 20th century, high in calories and low in physical activity, their genetic makeup left them "unprotected" from obesity and diabetes.

Here are some things you can't blame for directly causing your type II diabetes: the flu or any other illness, stress, being around someone who has diabetes, or something in particular you ate.

Today, we exercise less frequently than we should and often eat an unbalanced diet. We eat foods that are high in fat and refined sugar, while we tend to eat few slowly digestible starchy foods (complex carbohydrates) and little fiber. The way we live—high in calories and low in exercise—is probably the main reason that type II diabetes is so common.

HOW YOUR DIABETES WAS DISCOVERED

First, your doctor determined that you fit into the group of patients who are at high risk for diabetes. They are:

- Men and women with a family history of diabetes.

- Men and women who are obese.

- Women with a history of babies weighing more than 9 pounds at birth.

- Women who were diagnosed with temporary diabetes while pregnant (known as gestational diabetes).

- Men and women with high blood pressure or very high blood fat levels.

- Men and women with recurring skin, genital, or urinary tract infections.

Because diabetes is a disease in which your body's ability to remove glucose from your blood and deliver it to your cells is impaired, measuring the concentration of glucose in the blood is used to screen for diabetes. Your doctor took a blood sample at least three hours after your last meal. Under these conditions, a blood glucose measurement of 60 to 120 mg/dl (milligrams per deciliter) is usually found in people without diabetes. If the blood glucose level is 200 mg/dl or greater and the classic signs and symptoms of diabetes described above are seen, diabetes is the diagnosis. However, if the classic symptoms of diabetes are missing, more testing is needed to diagnose diabetes. The next step is to measure blood glucose levels twice when no food has been eaten for 10 to 12 hours. Fasting plasma glucose levels less than 115 mg/dl are considered normal. If both samples show a glucose level 140 mg/dl or greater, the diagnosis is diabetes.

4

> ### LIFE AFTER DIAGNOSIS
>
> For 44 years, I lived a normal, healthy life. It never once occurred to me that my family and I might have to face a completely different lifestyle. But on April 1, 1979, my medical problems, and our medical education, began.
>
> My diabetes went undiagnosed for several years as I battled bouts of vomiting and diarrhea. My digestive problems became increasingly worse. By late October 1983, I had lost 30 pounds and was physically exhausted.
>
> On December 26, the doctor told me to skip breakfast the next morning and report to the hospital lab at 8 AM for blood work.
>
> At 11:30 AM on the 27th the doctor arrived in the lab waiting room with the worst news I could imagine. My blood glucose was 460—almost four times the normal of 80–120. I had only a vague idea what the statement, "You have type II diabetes" meant. Little did I know then that this was actually good news.
>
> —*Carl M. Ward, Harrisonburg, Virginia*

Problems in interpreting fasting blood glucose results arise when the results are not clearly normal or abnormal. If this occurred, you might have been asked to take an oral glucose tolerance test. This test involves an overnight fast, followed by drinking 75 grams of glucose in the form of a sweet liquid. Blood samples are taken at specific times after consuming the drink. Test results from a person without diabetes show blood glucose levels rising rapidly, then falling below 140 mg/dl within two hours as insulin goes to work clearing glucose from the blood. If this test was used in your diagnosis of diabetes, your blood glucose levels were above 200 mg/dl one and two hours after consuming the glucose drink.

When the blood glucose response is in between normal and diabetic, a diagnosis of impaired glucose tolerance can be given. People with impaired glucose tolerance do not have diabetes. On retesting, up to 50 percent of people with impaired glucose tolerance have normal responses. However, if overweight, people with impaired glucose tolerance can develop type II diabetes later in life. They may be able to stop any further progression toward type II diabetes by weight loss and exercise.

How Your Body Changed

Type II diabetes is not a simple disease. You can't finger the one thing that went wrong that caused your diabetes to appear when it did, because it probably wasn't just one thing. To understand what type II diabetes is, you need to know something about diabetes in general.

Removing the pancreas from an animal brings on diabetes. Injecting insulin keeps the animal healthy. This is because the pancreas is the source of the insulin in the body. Insulin is a protein, which is made up of smaller molecules called amino acids. Insulin is produced and released (a process known as secretion) by cells in the pancreas called beta cells. Beta cells are found in groups called islets of Langerhans (named after their discoverer). With each meal, insulin is released and helps the body use or store the glucose generated from food.

If the beta cells in the islets die, insulin is no longer produced. In people with type I diabetes, all or most of the beta cells have ceased to function as a result of destruction by their body's immune system. This is an example of an immune system mechanism that has gone awry. These people depend on injected insulin to keep healthy, and type I diabetes is called insulin-dependent diabetes.

In contrast, people with type II diabetes do not lose the ability to make insulin. Instead of having no insulin, most people with type II diabetes show signs of insulin resistance— their bodies resist the successful action of insulin. Areas that accept insulin, called receptors, are found on the surface of cells that use glucose for energy, such as muscles. Insulin must combine with its receptor for glucose to enter the cell. In some people with type II diabetes, there are not enough insulin receptors on the surfaces of cells or the insulin receptors are abnormal, so blood levels of both insulin and glucose remain high. In most people with type II diabetes, the problem lies inside the cell, such that insulin cannot work properly even after combining with its receptor. (In rare cases, the insulin that is secreted is not built correctly and cannot be used or it does not fit into the insulin receptor.) These problems are examples of insulin resistance.

Many people with type II diabetes also have reduced levels of insulin secretion because their beta cells are not functioning well. This means that there is not enough insulin secreted to meet the body's needs, and this also results in high levels of glucose in the blood. It's unknown why insulin secretion is too low in many people with type II diabetes. One theory is that the mechanism that senses glucose levels and then tells the pancreas to secrete insulin does not work well. Another possibility is that after many years (perhaps decades) of insulin overproduction to combat insulin resistance, the pancreas simply begins to "burn out."

By now you should be getting an idea of how complicated type II diabetes is. Your doctor will try different treatments to assist your body in coping with diabetes. If a particular treatment is successful, your doctor may even be able to figure out which of the many causes of type II diabetes are at work in your body. With treatment, people can control type II diabetes (many are reversing their diabetic state by lowering their insulin resistance) and lead full and healthy lives. Even so, there is no cure. It's up to you to make the decision to achieve good health and good diabetes control.

Why Good Diabetes Control Makes Good Sense

For years, type II diabetes was not taken seriously. In fact, it was once referred to as a "touch of sugar" or "mild" diabetes because the symptoms are usually so subtle. Unlike type I diabetes, which tends to strike children and young adults and can kill swiftly if not treated with insulin, the so-called "other" diabetes creeps up slowly usually in our middle years, often with very vague or no symptoms; type II diabetes, if left untreated, just kills more slowly. (Just as type I diabetes can appear in adults, type II diabetes sometimes appears in young people, especially in American Indians. Studies have shown that young relatives of people with type II diabetes often show higher than normal insulin resistance; obesity and diabetes follow in later years.)

However, the term "mild" does not apply. Untreated type II diabetes can easily lead to complications that affect the heart, blood vessels and circulation, nerves, kidneys, and eyes. In fact, one of the particular dangers of type II diabetes is that it does develop slowly and sometimes is not readily recognized. Often, its symptoms are viewed as part of (or an acceleration of) the aging process and, so, are dismissed. Years of undiagnosed diabetes means that the damage of diabetes complications may have been building. Therefore, it is very important to take control of diabetes right from the first day of diagnosis.

HAVING DIABETES CAN MAKE YOU HEALTHIER

Five years after his diagnosis of type II diabetes when he was in his mid-50s, jazz trumpeter Red Rodney boasted that he was healthier than he'd ever been in his life.

Red discovered he had diabetes when he had a hypoglycemic episode on stage in Toronto, Canada. "I got dizzy—I really felt faint. I was leaning against the piano, and I was lost. I didn't know where I was in the tune...I could hear the chittering in the audience—they thought I was drunk. Finally, a lady in the audience came up on the bandstand and gave me a cracker and told me to eat it immediately. I did and came around." The woman explained to Red that her husband had diabetes and that she carried the crackers for him. When Red got home, he went to his doctor, and the diagnosis was diabetes.

To control his diabetes, Red had to make some changes in his lifestyle. For instance, Red never exercised before he was diagnosed. Now he swims or works out with an exercise tape or on an exercise bike, and he has a membership in a national health club so that he can exercise while on the road.

He also watches his diet, which hasn't been too difficult except when he's on the road, where sometimes it is hard to find something to eat when he needs it. "I

(Cont.)

(Cont.)

have to prepare for that because you expend a lot of energy playing an hour-and-a-half concert, and if you take your insulin, you must eat something after that. I'm always looking for places or bringing something I can have after the concert."

At first, Red took only oral diabetes medication. But a year later, his doctor wanted to put him on insulin. The thought frightened Red until he was converted while in the hospital for a minor operation. "When you are in the hospital they put you on insulin automatically, which was very lucky for me because I saw how well controlled my diabetes was during that period. When I came out of the hospital, it was easy."

"...I know so many people, when they find out they have diabetes, feel it is the end of the world. It's not. We can live normally, maybe even better than normal, if we stay in control. I certainly don't live a normal life, but look at me—I'm healthier than ever."

Having regular medical checkups and maintaining good control of your blood glucose levels are the best things you can do to stop the damage of diabetes complications. It's important to know the complications that may be caused by years of undetected high glucose levels:

- **Eyes:** people with diabetes may get diabetic retinopathy. In this process, small blood vessels in the eyes leak or break and cause tissue damage. It can lead to blindness.

- **Heart and blood vessels:** people with diabetes have a greater incidence of heart and blood vessel disease, especially heart attacks and strokes. Atherosclerosis (hardening of the arteries) can occur at an earlier age and advance more quickly. Small blood vessels (in the eyes, kidneys, and feet) can also be affected.

- **Kidneys:** people with diabetes have more kidney abnormalities and bladder infections. After a number of years, the kidney may show signs of tissue damage and fail to function.

- **Nerves:** people with diabetes can develop nerve damage, called neuropathy. It can affect nerves that make your muscles move, nerves that help you sense your surroundings or pleasure or discomfort, and nerves that control your unconscious functions, such as the beating of the heart and digestion. Neuropathy can be responsible for burning, tingling, or numbness in the hands, legs, or feet and an inability to differentiate between hot and cold. It's possible for nerve damage to result in painless heart attacks, dizziness, double vision, ringing or buzzing in the ears, an inability to digest food, constipation, diarrhea, nausea, and gas. Men may experience impotence; women may suffer from decreased sexual arousal or dry vaginal walls.

TAKING CARE OF YOUR HEALTH

The key to good diabetes control is **balance**. Good control means keeping blood glucose levels as near to normal as safely possible. Diet, exercise, and insulin or prescribed oral diabetes medications each play a role in controlling your blood glucose level.

The first and most important thing to do for your good health is lose weight if you need to. The severity of type II diabetes can be dramatically lessened by reaching and maintaining your healthy body weight; even a modest weight loss can help. A lifestyle built around a low-fat, well-rounded diet and regular exercise will enable you to control your body weight and reduces insulin resistance.

If you take insulin or oral diabetes medication, you need to match the doses with the amount of food you eat. If you eat more food than your medicine can handle, your blood glucose level will become too high. However, if you don't eat enough food, your blood glucose level can become too low. You will need a meal plan to follow daily that is created just for you. The medication you take and the foods you eat also need to match your activity pattern. So, your meal plan may include a snack before your scheduled exercise. Or, if an activity that wasn't planned comes up, you may need to eat a snack before or during your exercise session.

It's also important that you and your doctor make regular adjustments in your diabetes care program if needed to help you keep this balance. Your need for medication will probably change as you lose (or gain) weight and as you grow older.

Reaching a perfect balance and keeping it all the time is nearly impossible. However, with some effort, planning, motivation, and guidance, you can keep your diabetes in acceptable control. And that's a great investment in your good health.

Recognizing Your Feelings

If you've just been diagnosed with type II diabetes, it will take time to absorb all the information and instructions your health-care professionals will provide to you. It also will take your family some time to adjust. Maybe you've known about your diabetes for some time but weren't ready to face it.

"Why me?" many people ask. "It's so unfair!" "I'm angry. I don't want this disease. I don't want to treat it. I don't want to control it. I hate it!"

Diabetes can make us feel threatened. The diagnosis can bring fear of insulin injections, insulin reactions, comas, and future complications. Living with diabetes means lifestyle changes—eating less of foods we love, following a treatment schedule, monitoring blood glucose levels—that can threaten our self-esteem. It is natural to feel angry about having diabetes.

Your reaction to the diagnosis of diabetes may have been disbelief. "I don't have that disease." Or, "I have only a little diabetes." We may lessen the threat by believing we have something else—maybe something that losing a few pounds will cure. Even when we seem to accept that we have diabetes, our behavior may not reflect our acceptance.

We may make light of the disease and rob ourselves of the chance to grieve for some of what we've lost. Each of us wants to believe that we are perfect, immortal, and able to live our lives exactly how we choose. But, at some point, we all need to face and accept our limitations.

Yet, even when we do accept our limitations, we do not always want to follow meal plans and exercise regimens. Making the decision that we deserve to do all we can to be in good health takes some of us longer than others. It often means weighing the benefits of an immediate, concrete pleasure like food against a long-term, less defined reward like better health. Why does our determination fail us?

Here are some reasons cited by many people with diabetes.

"I'm afraid of what people will think."

"I don't want pity."

"Diabetes? Not me." "I won't be liked." "I will be teased."

"I don't want to be different."

"I won't be successful if I admit I have diabetes."

"Diabetes is ruining my life."

Keep in mind that there is an emotional element in diabetes. The diagnosis itself, the daily management of this chronic disease, your feelings of vulnerability, and your fears of the future can work together to create resentment, anger, and anxiety. Those feelings may, in turn, affect diabetes control.

The many feelings we have about our diabetes will never leave us completely. We need to accept the recurring episodes of anger and resentment. The bright side is that as we learn more about how we feel, we become better at recognizing our feelings as they occur. Instead of treating ourself like a failure for having negative feelings or reaching out for help, we can take comfort in knowing that our feelings are a normal part of having a chronic disease.

Having diabetes changes our life in positive ways. Diabetes increases our negotiating skills. We learn to make decisions about trading one food for another. We learn that a little less body weight or a little more exercise means less medication and more freedom. Having diabetes means acquiring discipline. Discipline can spill over into other aspects of our life: patience with our family, commitment in our work. Diabetes requires acceptance, accepting our limitations and those of others.

The longer we have diabetes, the easier some parts become. But new challenges will pop up. Some self-care tasks become more difficult. Like life, diabetes is a journey of self-discovery with no set finish line.

COPING WITH DIABETES

Coping strategies that work for you and your family will depend on the issues diabetes is raising and your family's coping style. Although none of these strategies may fit your

11

DENIAL AND ACCEPTANCE

Am I the only one who reads all the material on diabetes and has a hard time retaining it? I reject what I read—it doesn't apply to me. Those side effects won't happen to me. I don't feel any different. Why should I have to prick my finger so many times a day and drop blood on a strip? Why should I care if the numbers read 80 or 400? I don't feel *any* different. What does it matter if I vegetate or if I exercise?

Why should I have diabetes? I don't want it. It never lets up; it never goes away—it is constant. It affects no one but myself, and I'm the one who must handle the problems. Even as I think these things, I know them to be self-pitying and self-destructive.

I don't have the answers. What I do have are many unresolved feelings about type II diabetes. The diet, medication, and constant monitoring are overwhelming. I'm new at this, and I'm still in a state of shock and confusion.

I struggle with acceptance, with understanding, and with my motivation. I read articles that say, "It took me two, three, four years to accept the responsibility for my own diabetic health care."

I read, "I hate being diabetic, but find that I can live with it."

Nowhere do I read how to arrive at a point of acceptance, how to gain understanding, how to live with diabetes. I am at a point where I have awareness but not commitment, knowledge but not understanding, diabetes but not acceptance.

It's time for me to know I have diabetes. It's time for me to care.

—*Mary J. Eno, Melrose, Massachusetts*

situation, they might help you develop your own solutions.

- **Educate people about diabetes**. Instead of worrying about what people think about diabetes, take the initiative. Explain to them just what it means to have diabetes. You'll find they're interested and supportive.

- **Keep your privacy, if you prefer.** You decide what to tell friends and how much. Be sure your family knows to follow your guidelines. However, remember that you may need help in situations like low blood glucose reactions. Each time you are open about your diabetes with someone new, you reaffirm your own acceptance that you live each day with diabetes.

- **Keep the lines of communication open.** Sometimes talking is the best answer. On days when you've had a problem, talk to your friends or family. You may find this calms you down and is a much better choice than eating too much.

- **Keep a sense of humor.** Turn a negative situation into a positive one by looking for the lighter side!

- **Therapy may help you accept that you have diabetes.** In therapy, you can learn to help yourself, rather than denying the disease.

Everyone's life presents challenges—ours is living well with diabetes. Most of us are struggling with our own private reasons for not wanting to follow our diabetes treatment program. Part of taking care of ourselves is devising strategies with the help of our families, friends, and health-care professionals for healthy living.

On the surface, it seems simple. We have diabetes. We learn what to do to take care of ourselves, then we do what we need to do.

Sticking with a diabetes treatment regimen is rarely easy. For you, it may first take accepting that you have this disease and then making the decision to "happily" live with it. Picture yourself living a healthy, satisfying life with diabetes.

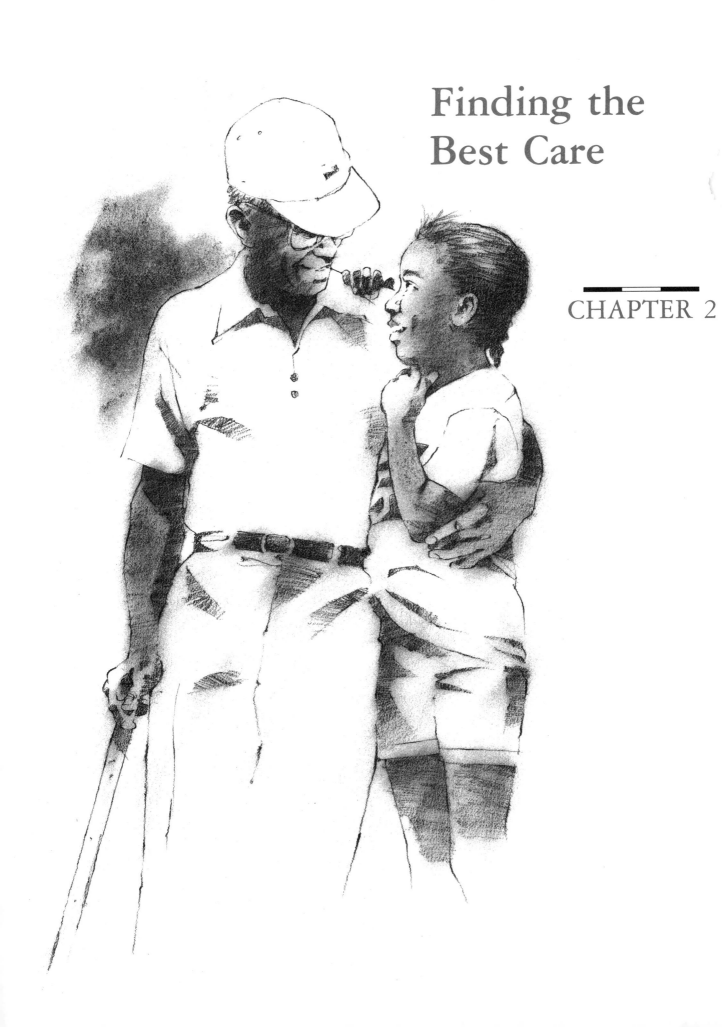

Finding the
Best Care

CHAPTER 2

For anyone with diabetes, finding the best possible care is a major concern. An important part of getting good care is becoming an educated medical consumer.

This means taking an active role in managing your diabetes, staying up-to-date on changes in diabetes care, asking questions of your health-care professionals, and taking advantage of the resources in your community. Overwhelmed? You needn't be. You don't have to face this alone. Here are some guidelines, suggested resources, and general help in arranging the best care possible for yourself. Finding the best care begins with you.

WHERE TO START

Diabetes is not a simple disease to manage. You'll want to find medical care that includes special knowledge and experience in dealing with diabetes. What should this care include? Who is qualified to provide it? How do you go about getting it? The American Diabetes Association has published specific recommendations concerning the standards of medical care that people with diabetes should have and who should provide it. The information in this chapter is drawn from these ADA guidelines.

The goal of your care should be to live well with diabetes and to help avoid short-term complications such as too high or too low blood glucose levels and long-term complications such as eye disease (retinopathy), nerve damage (neuropathy), or kidney disease (nephropathy). Achieving this goal involves many aspects of your everyday life—what you eat, the type of exercise you do, and any medications your doctor prescribes. Because diabetes is many different diseases, no one treatment plan works for everyone. The best care includes an **individual** plan tailored to your specific problems and needs. This plan will fit your lifestyle and eating habits to the greatest extent possible. Refining this plan may take time as you and your health-care professionals come up with a workable, livable routine. As that routine changes, so will your plan.

Your health-care options in striving for this goal may be intimately connected with your health insurance coverage. Many aspects of your care options depend on your selection of a health insurance plan. And, in turn, your selection of a plan may hinge on what you perceive your health-care needs to be.

This chapter includes a section on health insurance concerns for people with diabetes. It will help you sort out the kind of care you should receive, ideally who should provide it, and resources for locating it.

ASSEMBLING YOUR HEALTH-CARE TEAM

In recent years, the trend in diabetes care has been toward the **team** approach. Creating a health-care team is one of the most important things you can do to care for your type II diabetes. This approach acknowledges the fact that diabetes affects many aspects of your life each day and that there are health-care professionals who specialize in these areas, such as diet and medication, exercise, and diabetes complications, who should coordinate your care.

You are the most important member of your health-care team. You do the exercising, you make and eat the good foods on your meal plan, you must carefully administer your medication, and you must monitor the results. You are the first to notice any problems. You must take action if you need help. All team members will rely on you to communicate to them the information you learn about your body and its responses to diabetes.

The rest of the team includes your mate and family, your primary care physician (internist, family practice physician, or endocrinologist), diabetes educator (who is often a nurse), dietitian, and other health-care professionals as needed, such as an eye specialist, podiatrist, social worker/psychologist/psychiatrist, and exercise physiologist. The primary care physician should serve as your main source of diabetes care.

Sometimes these professionals will already be assembled as a team in a medical setting that specializes in diabetes care. Otherwise, you may have to assemble your own group or come as close to it as you can. It is well worth the effort. Ask your primary care physician to suggest a diabetes educator or dietitian to help you work out your treatment plan if your doctor doesn't have such a person on the staff. Anyone with diabetes who has established good communication with a dietitian or diabetes educator will tell you of its benefit. Ask your primary care physician for referrals to other medical specialists you may want to include on your health-care team.

17

YOUR PRIMARY CARE PHYSICIAN

Your primary care physician serves as the coordinator of your health-care team and is your main source of care. Ideally, you may want a doctor with expertise and special interest in diabetes. A doctor of internal medicine who has obtained additional years of study (and usually certification) in diseases such as diabetes is called an endocrinologist and can serve as your primary care physician. If you are searching for a new physician, check with friends or relatives who have diabetes and are satisfied with their medical care, ask your local ADA chapter for recommendations, get referrals from a physician you know and trust, or try your local hospital's or a physician's professional society's doctor referral service (see Resources). When selecting a new physician, consider

- Who is available in your area?

- What are their credentials? Ask about board certification in endocrinology and internal medicine and membership in professional associations such as the ADA, the Endocrine Society, or the American College of Physicians.

- Is your particular health insurance accepted for payments?

If you are thinking about joining a Health Maintenance Organization (HMO) or other type of prepaid health insurance plan, you may be required to use certain participating physicians. There is no harm in asking these physicians about their interest and expertise as you decide who to see. There is more on evaluating your options under various health insurance plans later in this chapter.

If possible, schedule an appointment just to talk with the doctor. Some health-care professionals charge for this time, so be sure to ask whether there will be an "interview" fee. During the interview, take time to look over the office. Is the staff polite? How long are you kept waiting past your appointment time? Are educational materials on display?

When you meet with the doctor, you may want to ask the following questions. Write them down ahead of time, and don't be shy about referring to your list during the interview.

- What percentage of your patients have diabetes? Are there more type I or type II diabetic patients? How many patients like me do you see a month?

- How often will regular visits be scheduled? How often will you check my glycosylated hemoglobin (see Chapter 3) and feet?

- Who covers for you on your days off?

- What procedures should be followed in the event of an emergency?

- Are you associated with other health-care professionals so that I can benefit from a team approach?

GETTING THE MOST FROM YOUR VISIT

Advance preparation can help you get the most from your trip to the doctor's office. If you're switching to a new doctor:

- Check to see.that your medical records have arrived at the new physician's office.

- Prepare a family medical history, including cause of parent's or sibling's death, and specific illnesses in family, such as hypertension (high blood pressure), coronary artery disease, and strokes.

- Write down the types of foods you eat for breakfast, lunch, dinner, and snacks.

- List any exercise you do.

- Bring a record of your blood glucose levels if you do self-monitoring.

- Bring all your medications. Prepare a list of any medications you currently take, including dosage.

- Prepare a list of questions for the doctor.

- Wear easy-to-remove clothes and footwear; you will probably need to undress for the physical exam.

Evaluating your interview is just as important as asking the right questions during it. How did it feel? Did the doctor seem genuinely concerned about you and your health goals? Did you feel free to speak up? Did you feel like you were heard?

CAN WE TALK?

Communication doesn't always comes easily. This can be especially true when you're feeling nervous, worried, or under pressure. Here are some tips for smooth communication between you and your health-care professional:

- Share the conversation. Your doctor should talk about 60 percent of the time, you should talk about 40 percent. Although it's important to speak up, it's also important to listen to what the doctor has to say.

- If the vocabulary becomes too technical and you don't understand, interrupt. Ask for an explanation.

- Ask your doctor to repeat anything you don't understand. Don't hesitate to take the time to write down information or instructions.

- Don't be afraid to bring up sexual or personal topics.

- Don't be afraid to discuss money. Compassionate health-care practitioners realize that financial worries can increase a patient's anxiety, and most should discuss payment options.

- Consider bringing a support person (spouse or relative) to sit in on the visit.

GETTING PHYSICAL

Once you've decided who will be your primary care physician, you will want to schedule a complete physical. Your first visit will also include giving your medical history. If this is the first time you have met your new primary care physician, take time for a get-acquainted talk. This is a good opportunity to evaluate how the doctor listens to you. Does the doctor seems genuinely concerned about your diabetes control and experienced with diabetic patients? Are questions answered to your satisfaction? Is the doctor listening? Does the doctor seem understanding? If you are struggling to lose weight, criticism and accusations won't help. An understanding physician can make a big difference. The object is to find competent care and health-care professionals with whom you are comfortable.

Complete physical exams are important for everyone but especially important for people with diabetes. The unpleasant facts are that diabetes puts you at greater risk for developing diabetic complications involving the eyes, kidneys, nervous system, heart, and circulatory system. You are also at increased risk for infections. This will be of no surprise to you if your diabetes was diagnosed during a visit to the doctor for treatment of one of these complications.

By taking charge of your health and seeking the best care possible, you can help turn the odds in your favor. Regularly scheduled physical exams are your first line of defense and an important part of getting the best possible care for your diabetes. Most complications begin as very small problems, unnoticeable on your part. Your health-care professionals are trained and equipped to notice early warning signs. Regular checkups help your primary care physician detect problems as early as possible.

YOUR MEDICAL HISTORY

If you're seeing a primary care physician or other health-care professional for the first time or if you're newly diagnosed with type II diabetes, be prepared to provide your medical history. Although the forms used to record your medical history vary from one health-care professional to the next, all will want to know the answers to certain questions. A lot of the questions are on matters that are private; answer honestly, and be assured that your health-care professional will maintain confidentiality. Open, honest communication is the basis for quality health care.

A lot of the information may be hard to recall correctly. When you make your appointment, ask for the history form to be mailed to you in advance of your visit so you can work on it at your leisure. Then take it with you to your appointment. The more complete and correct the picture you provide, the better your health care.

(Cont.)

22

(Cont.)

Most histories include questions about the health of your close relatives. Think about the general health and specific diseases found in your family, especially your mother, father, grandparents, and brothers and sisters. You will also be asked to give a general inventory of past and present health problems, such as back pain, appendicitis, frequent headaches, and depression. Do not hide or deny illnesses such as psychiatric disorders or AIDS.

Dig out your record of immunizations. You may even need to call past health-care providers for dates and names of procedures. Here are just a few health-related questions you'll probably be asked:

- What medications are you taking?

- Do you smoke? Have you ever smoked? If so, how much and for how long?

- Do you have any allergies?

- Have you ever been pregnant? What was the outcome?

- When were your last chest X ray, eye exam, and dental exam?

- Have you ever been treated by a psychiatrist?

- Have you recently lost or gained weight? What was your maximum weight? What did you weight at diagnosis of diabetes?

- Have you ever been rejected for health insurance or employment for a medical reason?

- Do you use any street drugs?

Some of these questions will be difficult to answer. You may not remember, or you may not want to be reminded. Make an attempt to overcome your fears of being judged harshly by what you put on the form. A concerned health-care professional will use this information to provide you with the best possible care, not to criticize you. Your good health is what it's all about.

If you have diabetes and are over age 30, the ADA recommends that you have a comprehensive physical exam once a year. (If you are over age 30, you should also have a complete eye and vision exam by an eye doctor annually.) Note that your primary care physician may want you to have a complete checkup more often if your diabetes is not well controlled or to monitor complications. For more on what tests to expect during regular visits and a complete physical, see Chapter 3.

THE REST OF YOUR HEALTH-CARE TEAM

A nurse educator or **diabetes nurse practitioner** is a registered nurse (RN) with special training and experience in caring for people with diabetes. Nurse educators may teach— explaining what diabetes is, how to use diabetes medications (or insulin), how to self-monitor blood glucose levels, and how to handle sick days and pregnancy. The initials CDE (certified diabetes educator) indicate that the nurse has passed a national qualifying exam in diabetes education.

A dietitian is a health-care professional with training and expertise in the field of nutrition. A dietitian is the professional best suited to help you develop and modify your meal plan—a crucial component to living well with diabetes. Look for the initials RD (registered dietitian), which indicate that the dietitian has passed a national credentialing exam. Many states also require a license, so you'll often see the initials LD (licensed dietitian). Some dietitians are also CDEs. Ask whether they are members of the ADA or The American Dietetic Association.

An eye doctor (optometrist or ophthalmologist) is an especially important member of the health-care team. Your eye-care specialist monitors the changes in your eyes, particularly those associated with diabetes, and determines what those changes mean and how to treat them or when to refer you to another eye specialist. Your eye doctor should be familiar with diabetic retinopathy, laser therapy, and vitrectomy. Also ask your eye-care specialist

- What percentage of your patients have diabetes?

- Do you perform eye surgery? (This is usually limited to ophthalmologists.)

- Are you a retina specialist? (This is important because diabetic eye disease affects the retina, the light-sensitive cells at the back of the eye that help form visual images.)

- Will you send regular reports to my primary care physician?

The ADA recommends yearly eye exams.

Social worker/psychologists/psychiatrists are the healthcare professionals trained to help with the personal and emotional aspects of diabetes management. Social workers must have a master's degree in social work (MSW) as well as training in individual, group, and family therapy. The initials LCSW indicate a licensed clinical social worker who has passed a state credentialing exam. Social workers can help you cope with a variety of issues, from psychosocial problems relating to diabetes control in family or work situations to locating community or government resources to help with medical or financial needs.

A clinical psychologist who works directly with patients can have a master's or doctorate degree in psychology and is trained in individual, group, and family psychology. You might visit a psychologist during a particularly stressful few weeks or months for short-term help or on a long-term basis to work out more deep-seated problems.

A psychiatrist is an MD who is able to prescribe medications and advise hospitalization for emotional disturbances.

A podiatrist is trained to treat foot and related lower-extremity disorders. Podiatrists graduate from a college of podiatry with a Doctor of Podiatric Medicine (DPM) degree and have completed a residency in podiatry.

Foot care is especially important for you. This is because people with diabetes are highly susceptible to poor blood circulation and nerve disease in the extremities—on top of a tendency to develop infections. Sores, even small ones, can turn into serious problems quickly. Any foot sore or callus should be checked by your primary care physician or a podiatrist. Don't try fixing these yourself.

Podiatrists treat corns, calluses, or foot sores so as to prevent more serious problems. They demonstrate the correct way to cut toenails and how to buy properly fitting shoes. To find a podiatrist, check with your primary care physician, area

THE PAINLESS HURT

The trouble with diabetes is that it doesn't hurt. If a pain had shot through my side every time my blood glucose rose above 150 mg/dl, you can bet I would have maintained good control over my diabetes. But the problem is that it doesn't hurt until it's too late.

At the age of 25 in 1974, I was diagnosed, in the terms of that era, as "borderline diabetic." Nowadays, we know that you either are or you aren't. Knowing only that diabetes had something to do with sugar, I asked the doctor exactly what diabetes was. He pulled a large medical encyclopedia off his shelf, literally tossed it to me, and said, "Look it up." Then he left the room.

Needless to say, I did not control my diabetes. What for? The excessive urination and thirst was just a minor inconvenience. "I'll just keep taking the pills, and that'll take care of it," I told myself.

By 1986, I was a lot older, but not a lot wiser. I was already showing symptoms of diabetes-related complications. For about three months I monitored my health well. But high blood glucose readings easily discouraged me. Stress, bad news, good news, a cold, tough day at the office—the facts of life—all contributed to my soaring blood glucose levels. Because of this and the fact I was reassigned to a doctor in my health maintenance organization who had a three-month waiting list, I let my control slide. If I had insisted on better care, maybe I could have avoided some of the health problems I developed.

After a while, I reached the point where I knew when I was going to have a high blood glucose reading, so I solved the problem. I quit testing. Brilliant. Like the man who read so much about the bad effects of smoking that he gave up reading, I gave up testing and reading about diabetes. I even let my membership in the American Diabetes Association expire. It was only an annoying reminder of my silent curse.

At the age of 40, I was so out of control I finally had to start insulin therapy. I was seen only by a physician's

(Cont.)

(Cont.)

assistant. The doctor who wrote the prescription and authorized refills never saw me. I could have had three legs, and he wouldn't have known. There was no follow-up or monitoring. I was negligent for not demanding to see the doctor until it was too late.

In April 1990, I had a three-week bout of violent coughing and gasping for breath to the extent that I suffered headaches and back pains. Again, I did not demand the medical care I needed. One doctor finally determined that I had viral pneumonia and prescribed cough syrup. The next day, I had a stroke.

The relationship between the coughing and the stroke are a matter of medical opinion, but the relationship between diabetes and stroke are a medical fact. Lying in the hospital bed that first night—scared, angry, and guilt-ridden—I realized this disease of mine that hadn't hurt for so many years now hurt like hell.

I felt I was now paying the price for the years of eating junk because I had lost the ability to swallow. The stroke, although not totally debilitating, paralyzed the muscles on the left side of my face—including the mechanisms used to swallow—and the right side of my body.

Fortunately, my prognosis is good. Because I'm only 41 years old and I regained the ability to swallow much sooner than my doctor thought I would, I'm hopeful. I may even regain the feeling on my right side in a couple of years.

Have I learned my lesson? Will I have the willpower to stay away from the foods that I love, or at least monitor the quantities? Will I test my blood religiously? I think so. I hope so. God, I wish this disease had hurt before.

—*Steve Berk, Houston, Texas*

hospitals, or your local ADA chapter. During your initial visit, ask what percentage of the podiatrist's patients have diabetes.

At first it may seem odd to think of your **dentist** as a member of your health-care team. However, dentists play an important role by helping you maintain a healthy mouth and strong teeth. Because of the high risk of poor circulation and infections, people with diabetes are at a somewhat higher—and earlier—risk than people without diabetes for periodontitis, a form of gum disease. It's important to have regular dental checkups and to tell your dentist that you have diabetes.

An **exercise physiologist** is the person to enlist if you are thinking of adding exercise to your daily routine. Fitness programs are best designed by a person trained in the scientific basis of exercise and safe conditioning techniques. Look for someone who has a master's or doctorate degree in exercise physiology or for a licensed health-care professional who has had graduate training in exercise physiology. Another way you have of telling whether a health-care professional has the basic skills required to design a safe, effective fitness program for you is certification from an organization such as the American College of Sports Medicine.

Exercise physiologists can plan individual exercise programs that are tailored to your specific needs. Some examples include improving cardiovascular fitness, lowering blood glucose, losing weight, or developing muscle fitness and flexibility. There are exercises for you if you have arthritis, are very overweight, have complications of diabetes, or have been sedentary and want to become more active. Any exercise program should first be approved by your primary care physician.

ORGANIZING THE TEAM

Your physician may already use a team approach to diabetes care and be working with many or all of the health professionals described above. Some hospitals or medical centers have professional members who work together. Others recommend professionals in different locations who contact each other regularly about your care.

If you have no health-care team available, think about putting one together yourself. Start by discussing it with your primary care physician. Be sure to ask if there will be extra consultation costs. If so, find out whether your insurance covers them.

If you and your physician agree on this approach, give each health-care professional the name, phone number, fax number, and address of the others. Ask your health-care team to consult on your care when appropriate. It's particularly good to do this when specific issues arise that concern you or when you or they contemplate changes in your diabetes care or lifestyle. For example, each team member should know if you are starting a weight-loss diet, joining an aerobics program, or starting a new medication.

If these guidelines are inappropriate to your situation, you will have to decide how much of a health-care team you can build. You may need to be responsible for communicating your test results and treatment responses between the professionals. You may have to do some extra reading to keep informed on advances in diabetes care (try your state's ADA affiliate for resources).

MORE ABOUT DIETITIANS

If you are newly diagnosed or even if you've had diabetes for some time, you may never have worked with a dietitian. Diet is perhaps the most important component of living well with type II diabetes and just plain living well. Unfortunately, diet can also be one of the most frustrating and disheartening aspects of taking good care of yourself. Here are some of the ways a dietitian can help.

Dietitians can explain the importance of nutrition and meal planning in diabetes care. They can also help devise a meal plan with you that—within reason—will take into account your personal tastes and preferences.

Even if you have had diabetes for some time, a dietitian can make a difference. A meal plan that's appropriate at one stage of your life may not be appropriate 5 or 10 years later. Switching jobs, increasing or decreasing physical activity, gaining or losing weight, and developing other conditions such as hypertension are just a few of the ways in which changes in your everyday routine can affect your nutritional needs.

Another reason to see a dietitian regularly is that research in medicine and nutrition continually changes what we know about diabetes and how to live well with the disease. Good examples of this are the changes in the ADA's and The American Dietetic Association's recommendations about increasing the amount of complex carbohydrates and fiber and lowering fat and sodium intake in the nutritional management of diabetes during the last 10 years.

Perhaps you're having trouble with your meal plan because it interferes with family dining or because you just plain don't like it. Maybe your meal plan needs to be more personalized. A dietitian can help you change this. Other ways a dietitian can help:

- **Teaching:** dietitians show you how to read food labels, how to handle eating out in restaurants, how to make healthy food choices when grocery shopping, and how to safely incorporate some sugar into your diet, if you like.

- **Explaining:** dietitians explain how to use the ADA's *Exchange Lists for Meal Planning* or how to fit foreign or ethnic food favorites into your meal plan.

- **Reading and resources:** dietitians help you discover a range of nutritional resources, including cookbooks and reference material, for learning how to prepare healthy, delicious, satisfying meals.

Good sources of referrals to help you find a dietitian include

- Your primary care physician

- Area hospitals

- Your local ADA chapter.

In addition, many members of The American Dietetic Association with a special interest in diabetes have joined the Diabetes Care and Education Practice Group (DCEPG). The DCEPG network coordinator for your area can help you find dietitians who are members.

Consider asking the following questions when you're selecting a dietitian.

- What percentage of your clients have diabetes?

- Will you be able to work well with my primary care physician and nurse educator?

- What are the cost of your services? How can they be covered by my insurance plan?

Initially, your dietitian will do an assessment to help design your meal plan. This will include questions about your health, lifestyle, and diabetes management routine as well as any diets you've tried in the past. You may be asked to keep a one- to three-day food diary.

Your dietitian will help you determine your nutritional requirements and translate them into a specific plan to work toward your personal goals, for example, weight loss, fat and cholesterol control, or lowering sodium intake. With the

---

FAKING IT

Our family recently had its annual physical exams. The results have just come in. They prove, once again, that in the case of Mrs. Miller and myself, opposites attract. Because of that, some drastic changes have been made at our house.

We finally accept the fact that we must take care of our health. I'm proud to say that we have begun to do just that. Are we engaged in daily exercise? No way. Are we on strict diets? Forget it. What are we doing? We are reading the several armloads of diet and exercise books that we bought when we got our test results. You might say that we are reading ourselves to good health.

Our physicals established the fact that our household is a perfect example of the Jack Spratt syndrome. Sort of. My wife has high cholesterol and can eat no fat. I have diabetes and can eat no sweets. Half the diet books we bought are about lowering cholesterol. The other half tell how to lower blood glucose. If only we both had the same condition, we could have saved a fortune buying half as many books.

Books aren't he only things we have been reading to help ourselves to better health. We have also been reading food labels. We are in search of products that will allow us to eat all the things we enjoy without suffering the consequences.

We have found fat foods without fat and sweet foods without sugar. We have also found that we can eat these fake foods without guilt. Fake guilt or otherwise.

—*Larry Miller, Grass Valley, California*

---

dietitian's help you will be able to tailor your meal plan to your specific health situation and also work with any other health problems that may affect your diet, such as kidney disease, high blood pressure, or high cholesterol levels.

Dietitians are not magicians, however. Relearning a lifetime of eating habits takes time and patience. Within reason, a dietitian can follow your food preferences and work them into a meal plan that will taste good, help keep your blood glucose levels under control, and meet your other treatment goals.

You'll leave with a meal plan on paper that is then put to the test in your everyday life. Follow-up visits with the dietitian allow for progress checks and adjustments to your meal plan. Generally, assessment visits take about an hour to an hour and a half. Follow-up visits run about 15 to 30 minutes. The ADA advises you to have routine diet counseling. You should see a dietitian every 6 to 12 months.

Fees for nutrition counseling vary widely. Some insurers cover it; some do not. Before you make your initial appointment, check with your health insurance company about your coverage. If they will reimburse for nutrition care services, find out what kind of documentation they require. For example, they may need a letter from your primary care physician. Some HMOs include dietitian's services in their basic benefits package; some do not.

When you arrange your initial visit, ask the dietitian about the fee, number of expected visits, methods of payment, and reimbursement.

Medicare Part B covers services that are "incidental to physicians' professional services" but specifies that they must be provided by employees of the physician. Some primary care physicians have a dietitian on their staff. Reimbursement goes to the physician.

DIABETES EDUCATION PROGRAMS

In recent years we've learned more than ever about diabetes and how to live well with this chronic disease. An important tool for helping people keep up with the latest information and ideas about diabetes care is the diabetes education program. These programs vary widely. Some are inpatient hospital programs, some are classes offered to outpatients, and some are provided through private physician's offices.

Whether you've just been diagnosed or you've had diabetes for several years, there is probably a diabetes education program that will help.

Your doctor may suggest a specific program, or you may

want to do some research and find out what is available in your area. To learn about local programs, contact your ADA state affiliate (listed in the white pages of your phone book) or ask your local hospitals, the county or state department of health, or your primary care physician. Then you'll need to contact specific programs and ask for information so that you can compare what they have to offer.

Diabetes education programs that meet the rigorous standards for diabetes education developed by the National Diabetes Advisory Board can apply to receive ADA Recognition. The ADA's Recognition process assures you that a specific diabetes education program is a quality program. To achieve Recognition, all aspects of a diabetes education program receive thorough review and scrutiny. The ADA can tell you which programs have achieved Recognition in your area.

When you are looking for a diabetes education program, consider the following:

■ Has the program achieved Recognition from the ADA?

■ Is the program appropriate to your needs? Some programs offer general diabetes education. Others teach survival skills for those newly diagnosed. Some focus on adults with type I diabetes, and others focus on adults with type II diabetes. Are the program materials suited to your needs? For example, do you require large-print materials or foreign-language translations?

■ How is the program presented? Some subjects, such as self-monitoring of blood glucose or food portion control, are best taught through group sessions with lots of student participation. Other subjects are appropriate to a lecture-style class. Some programs offer one-on-one teaching. Others have small group classes or a combination of both.

■ What's included in the program? The National Diabetes Advisory Board's standards require that any diabetes education program be able to offer information on each of the following topics:

General facts

Psychological adjustment

Family involvement

Nutrition

Exercise

Medications

Relationship between nutrition, exercise, and medications

Self-monitoring of blood glucose

Hyperglycemia and hypoglycemia

Illness

Complications (prevention, treatment, and rehabilitation)

Hygiene

Benefits and responsibilities of care

Use of health-care systems

Community resources

All of these topics should be included in the total curriculum of a diabetes education program, but titles may vary from program to program.

- Is the program individualized? You should have a say in what you study. Programs should conduct some type of assessment of your needs and then allow you to negotiate what you'd like to have in your education program.

- Is there some type of evaluation process? At the start, does the program assess what you know about diabetes? Is there a final evaluation to see what you've learned and what you might change about your diabetes management as a result of the course?

- Are the instructors qualified? Health-care professionals should be teaching the courses. At least one of the instructors should be an RN or an RD. Other teachers might include physicians, social workers, psychologists, podiatrists, pharmacists, exercise specialists, and foot- and eye-care specialists. How many instructors are CDEs?

- Is the program convenient? Will all teachers be in one location or will you have to travel? Are there proper spaces for the classes? Does the time and location fit in your schedule? How often is the course offered? How long does it run? Is it flexible?

■ Are there take-home materials? Is there an extra charge for these?

■ Is someone on call, at least during business hours, whom you can contact with diabetes management questions that don't require a physician?

■ Is there follow-up? You can't learn everything at once. You need time to practice and to an opportunity to come back with questions. Do you go back periodically? Is there an advanced course you can take? Are there follow-up classes to reinforce what you've learned?

CDEs

Diabetes educators appear in a variety of health-care professions, including nursing, dietetics, medicine, pharmacy, podiatry, psychosocial counseling, and exercise physiology. These professionals are involved in some aspect of teaching or caring for people with diabetes. They may work in hospitals, clinics, diabetes centers, or private offices.

To become certified, diabetes educators must pass a test offered by the National Certification Board for Diabetes Educators (NCBDE)—an independent organization established by the American Association of Diabetes Educators.

When you see the initials CDE after a health-care professional's name, you know that the professional is specially trained and up-to-date in the care and treatment of people with diabetes. CDEs pass an objective exam covering physiology, pharmacology, monitoring, complications, psychological issues, and teaching-learning principles related to diabetes. In addition, CDEs must update their education by passing a recertification test every 5 years.

■ Are education and treatment integrated? Will there be communications between the program staff and your physician? Those responsible for the program should keep a written record of what you've studied and how well you've done in your courses. They should share that information with your physician.

■ How much does it cost? What does the price you pay cover? Some programs charge for a package that includes a series of classes and class materials, others charge per visit. Make sure you know what whether additional costs are involved, such as travel, overnight lodging, meals, and books. If it's appropriate, ask whether there's a charge for a family member or friend who wants to take the program with you.

■ Will insurance cover part or all of the cost? Some programs routinely get third-party reimbursement, others do not. Check with your insurer to find out whether reimbursement for educational services is contingent on a doctor's prescription for the diabetes education course as part of your treatment.

35

HEALTH INSURANCE

With today's spiraling health-care costs, health insurance is vital. Living with a chronic disease such as diabetes can be expensive, even with health insurance. Finding the best possible coverage is important not only to your pocketbook but to living well with diabetes. You'll want to find a plan that meets your needs and your budget.

You may have the option of joining a **group policy** through health insurance offered by your employer. Group policies are usually open to all employees, regardless of their medical condition (however, coverage by employers employing only a few people may require health screening and medical history). Your employer will often pay for most or all of the insurance premium for you. These policies may also cover your spouse and children for additional fees. Health care is considered a nontaxable expense, so you may have the fees you pay for health-care coverage for you and your dependents (if you pay anything) taken from your paycheck before taxes are calculated.

Before you start a new job, ask about "preexisting conditions" exclusion to health-care coverage. Some companies' policies will not cover your diabetes care until some amount of time has passed, for instance, 6 or 12 months. If appropriate, you may want to retain coverage under your former employers's policy during this waiting period (see below). Another option is to purchase temporary short-term health-care coverage to protect you during this time.

If you have a group policy through work and leave your job, you can retain you current group coverage under a federal law called Consolidated Omnibus Budget Reconciliation Act (COBRA). This law requires employers, under certain circumstances, to allow employees who are leaving their jobs to keep the same insurance policy at group rates and with the same coverage for up to 18 months after they leave. This legislation applies not only to employees but also to covered dependents. You will be responsible for paying for the coverage and may be charged up to 2 percent more than the rate the company was charging your employer. This is almost always less expensive than purchasing a new short-term policy.

If you are not eligible for any form of group insurance, finding an affordable **individual policy** can be difficult. Individual policies are contracts between individuals and an insurance company and take into consideration medical history. However, remember that because you have diabetes, health insurance is a necessity.

Still, you may have other insurance options under the law. If you are over 65, you are eligible for federal health insurance under **Medicare**. Medicare covers a portion of hospital bills, doctor fees, and other expenses, but you will still have to pay for a large portion of your bills. Medicare is a federal health insurance program that is administered by each state.

You can sign up for Medicare three months before the month of your 65th birthday. A few months before you reach 65, contact your local Social Security Administration office. You can find the address and phone number under the United States Government listing in your telephone book. Bring your birth certificate along when you apply.

Not everyone over age 65 can get Medicare. For example, some people who worked at state or local government jobs are not eligible for Medicare. Check with your local Social Security Administration office if you are unsure about coverage. About 10 percent of people getting Medicare are under age 65. They qualify because they are disabled and cannot work.

If you have a very low income, you might be eligible for **Medicaid**, a federal and state assistance program. Medicaid regulations vary from state to state, so you'll have to contact your state's Medicaid office to find out whether you qualify and what health expenses will be covered. A social worker can help you with this.

WHAT YOU SHOULD KNOW ABOUT YOUR HEALTH INSURANCE PLAN

Can you list everything that's covered by your health insurance? To be an informed consumer, you should be able to answer most of these questions.

- Are visits to your primary care physician covered? Is there any limit on how many? How much you will have to pay per visit?

- Does the plan reimburse for diabetes education?

- Does the plan cover medical equipment and supplies? If you inject insulin or self-monitor your blood glucose, this is important.

- Does the plan cover the services of a dietitian? Managing diet is critical for people with diabetes.

- What mental health benefits are covered? The services of a social worker or psychologist can help you through rough spots of living with diabetes.

- Does the plan cover the services of specialists, such as a podiatrist, eye doctor, or dentist, whose care is very important to people with diabetes?

- What medications are paid for? Is there a prescription plan to reduce costs? How often can prescriptions be refilled? Is there a copayment fee for each prescription?

- What kind of home health care (such as having a visiting nurse change bandages or administer intravenous medicines at home) coverage is included? Are there any limitations?

Certain states guarantee your right to health insurance. These states offer "pooled-risk" health insurance for those who cannot get group or individual coverage (see Resources). The cost of pooled-risk insurance varies widely among the states that offer it. Most try to keep it affordable by placing limits on the premium. The cost, however, is still likely to be higher than individual coverage.

Fee-for-Service Versus Prepaid Health Plans

Fee-for-service is the traditional type of health insurance. In this system, the insurance company agrees to pay for all or some of the medical care you receive in exchange for the premium you and/or your employer pay. In this pay-as-you-go system, the insurer pays for the service you receive from your choice of doctors or hospitals. Usually you pay a yearly deductible and a portion of the cost of a visit (the copayment). Most plans reimburse at 100 percent after an out-of-pocket expense limit is met.

A lot of health-care professionals expect you to pay the total fee at the time of service. You must then apply to your insurance company to receive your reimbursable expenses. However, ask whether the physician or hospital will accept "assignment" of benefits (wait for your insurance company to pay its share) and bill you for the remainder. Expect paperwork and the possibility of having to pay all expenses up front. The advantage is freedom of choice among a wide range of health-care professionals and area hospitals with whom they are affiliated. The disadvantage is that preventive health care, for example a mammogram or Pap smear, is usually not covered.

In **prepaid** health plans, you and/or your employer pay a fixed premium and you receive comprehensive health care, from routine office visits to hospitalization. Your cost is its lowest if you seek care from the network of participating physicians and hospitals. There is generally no deductible to satisfy or paperwork to do. You also will not be expected to pay out large sums of money for services, so you have better control over your budget should unexpected illness occur. You can usually see specialists if referred to them by your primary care physician and/or if the specialist also participates in the prepaid health plan (although exceptions are made). Your choice of hospitals is also limited should you require other than emergency hospitalization. Health Maintenance Organizations (HMOs) are the best known type of prepaid health plan.

HMOs usually create a full-service health center by hiring or contracting with health-care professionals to work in their buildings. You must usually see someone under contract to or employed by the HMO to receive prepaid health care. There is often a small copayment for each service. The HMO makes arrangements for coverage for sickness or accidents when you travel outside the HMO's service area.

FIGHTING BACK

When your health insurer denies your request for reimbursement, you can fight back. It's not an easy process, and you may not always win, but it may be worth the effort. Insurance policies are contracts and, like all contracts, are open to interpretation.

Durable Medical Equipment

If your policy covers durable medical equipment, it may be possible to get coverage for a blood glucose meter for self-monitoring of blood glucose as prescribed by your physician. You'll probably need to accompany your claim with a certificate from your physician stating that the equipment is "medically necessary."

Prescription Medications and/or Medical Supplies

If your policy covers these, you may be able to get coverage for lancets and test strips. Keep copies of every prescription written for you. Ask your physician to write prescriptions for supplies that are needed (such as syringes) to take prescription medications, such as insulin, even if they are sold over-the-counter. Get a prescription for each item if your physician suggests you monitor your blood glucose levels. The prescription should itemize the meter and/or type of strips and blood-letting devices. Even if the item does not need a prescription at the drug store, get one anyway. You may need it to support your you insurance claim.

How to Appeal

Under most states' regulations, insurance companies have a time limit in which to act on your claim. (Check with your state insurance commission, listed in Resources.) The company does not have to decide on your claim in

(Cont.)

39

> *(Cont.)*
>
> that set period, but it does have to let you know the status. If your claim is denied, the insurance company is supposed to explain the reasons. After a denial, direct a written request for an appeal to the insurance company's claims manager. Explain your appeal, include copies of supporting prescriptions and correspondence, and ask them to contact you or your physician by a specific date. If you don't hear from them or are denied again, consider taking your claim to small claims court.

Medicare and You

How Medicare Helps With Hospital Bills. Once you are enrolled in Medicare, the plan can help pay part of your hospital bill. Under Medicare Part A, you must pay the first portion of the bill. This payment is called the deductible. The deductible increases each year. It represents the average cost of a one-day stay in a hospital. In 1991, the deductible was $628; this amount increased to $652 for 1992. These amounts are charged for each spell of illness that requires hospitalization; if you have been out of the hospital for 60 days, your next visit would be considered a new spell of illness.

After that, Medicare pays the full cost of your first 60 days in the hospital. It pays for a semiprivate room and the cost of such things as nursing services, medical supplies, lab work, X rays, and medicines.

If you are still hospitalized after 60 days, Medicare keeps helping. But you must start paying part of the bill. This is called the copayment. If you are in the hospital for a total of more than 90 days, that is when you must start paying the entire bill. However, you can use up to 60 days of lifetime reserve coverage to keep your copayment at the same level as days 60 through 90. Once those 60 days are "spent," they cannot be renewed.

Medicare will not pay for long-term nursing home care. Medicare Part A can help pay for short-term "skilled nursing care." Many nursing homes do not provide what Medicare defines as "skilled nursing care." So Medicare will not approve or pay for most nursing homes. To find out whether a nursing home is approved by Medicare, check with your local Social Security Administration office or the nursing home itself.

Medicare may pay for some part-time skilled nursing care in your home (home health care). Check with your primary care physician for details. Also, Medicare will pay for hospice care for those who are terminally ill.

How Medicare Helps With Doctors' Bills. Medicare Part B can help pay for a portion of your doctors' bills. You make a monthly contribution (about $32 per month in 1992). People who receive Social Security will have this amount withheld from their monthly Social Security checks. There is also a yearly deductible of $100, which you must pay before Medicare benefits begin.

After the deductible is satisfied, Medicare will pay 80 percent of the approved cost. You must pay the remaining 20 percent. Ask your doctor whether he or she accepts the assignment of a Medicare claim. If they do, you will only need to pay out your 20% copayment, and the doctor will accept the rest of the payment directly from Medicare based on Medicare's estimate of the prevailing charge for that service. If your doctor does not take assignment of a Medicare claim, you can be charged up to 120% of the prevailing charge (but that's the legal limit). You also may have to pay the entire bill yourself and wait for Medicare to reimburse you for 80 percent.

How Medicare Helps With Diabetes Care Expenses. Under Part B, Medicare pays for some diabetes supplies.

- Medicare will pay 80 percent of the cost of blood glucose meters for people prescribed insulin, as well as for lancets, strips, and other supplies used with the meter. Medicare will pay for test strips only if you are using a meter. You must have a written prescription for all of these items, over-the-counter or not, from your doctor as well as a written statement from your doctor detailing your diagnosis, fluctuations in your blood glucose levels, and your recommended self-monitoring schedule. Make copies of these written statements; you must give a copy of it to your pharmacist for your Medicare claim to be submitted each time you purchase these supplies.

- Medicare will pay for diabetes outpatient education in some states if particular criteria are met, such as if the program is in a hospital, if the education is considered medically necessary (for example, the primary care physician should write a "prescription" for education), and if the facility and program provider are Medicare approved.

- Medicare will pay for foot care.
- Medicare will pay for laser treatment for diabetic retinopathy (eye disease) and for cataract surgery.
- Medicare will not pay for insulin or syringes.
- Medicare will not pay for insulin pumps.
- Medicare will not pay for outpatient nutrition counseling services or dietitian services in some states.
- Medicare will not pay for regular eye exams or for eyeglasses.

How Medigap Plans Help. To fill the gaps in your coverage, you can choose from many so-called "Medigap" plans that pick up some or most of the charges Medicare won't cover. Medigap plans are private health insurance. There are federal standards that insurance policies must meet in order to be called a Medicare supplement policy. Be sure to read the policy carefully and comparison shop before buying one of these plans.

The booklet *Guide to Health Insurance for People With Medicare*, written by the National Association of Insurance Commissioners and the Health Care Financing Administration of the Department of Health and Human Services, is updated every year and is available through any insurance company. Ask for it. It contains the federal standards for Medigap policies and general information about Medicare. A more detailed explanation of Medicare is available as *The Medicare Handbook* from any Social Security Administration office (see Resources if you prefer to write away for it).

IN THE HOSPITAL

No one likes to think about it. After all, hospital visits mean medical problems, which can range from relatively minor elective surgery to life-threatening emergencies. Once admitted to a hospital, you are no longer in charge. Suddenly, your regular routine is disrupted, and you may face a recovery period of days, weeks, or months.

But the fact is, taking time now to think about and plan for handling hospital visits will pay off. You can take steps that will help ensure yourself the best possible care—whether you face an emergency hospitalization or one for which you can plan.

Plan Ahead

Start by learning something about your local hospitals. Which ones accept your health insurance? Perhaps your primary-care physician has privileges only at certain area hospitals.

WHEN YOU'RE IN THE HOSPITAL

Here are some tips to follow while in the hospital. On admission,

- Make it clear to doctors and nurses that you have diabetes.

- Tell them what medications you are taking for diabetes and any other medications you are taking. It helps to write a list ahead of time of all your medications, how often you take them, and in what dosages.

- State clearly and explain allergies or other conditions, such as vomiting, that could affect the actions of medications.

- Speak up about other medical conditions you have, including diabetic complications. High blood pressure may require special treatment before and during surgery. Heart disease medications may require adjustment.

- Tell them about any frequent low blood glucose reactions. Bring your self-monitoring records with you.

- Tell them about your meal plan. Ask to see the hospital dietitian and explain what kind of diet you're on, including any special modifications such as low salt, low cholesterol, or low fat.

Basically, there are three types of hospitals: city or county hospitals; private, community hospitals; and hospitals that are teaching centers, usually affiliated with a medical school.

However, these types of hospitals are not mutually exclusive: county or private hospitals can also be affiliated teaching hospitals. To learn about the hospital's general reputation, as well as its reputation for treating people with diabetes, start by seeking the opinion of your primary care physician. Talk over with your doctor steps to take in the event of emergency hospitalization and agree on a hospital to use. Ask your doctor where he would send a member of his family. Or you can ask friends, neighbors, or relatives who've had recent hospital-izations. Other resources for determining the reputation of a local hospital are your ADA chapter or your diabetes support group.

Try to learn these important facts about a hospital you are considering using.

- Are there endocrinologists on the staff?

- Does the hospital have diabetes educators and dietitians with expertise in diabetes on the staff? Are they available to both inpatients and outpatients?

- Is there a diabetes education program within the hospital or affiliated with the hospital?

- What other types of support services are available to people with diabetes?

Ask your health insurance which hospital services they will cover. Also, many insurance companies require you to notify them in advance of any hospital service (except emergencies) so they can precertify your treatment.

Facing Surgery

When you're facing surgery, it's normal to feel apprehensive. The good news is that with good care, people with diabetes recover about as well as anyone. But blood glucose control can suffer around the time of an operation, and diabetes can complicate recovery and prolong your hospital stay unless the diabetes is closely managed. Take an active role in helping yourself recover on schedule by doing everything you can to have good diabetes control.

Emergency surgery aside, your first question may be whether or not the surgery is necessary. If a doctor recommends surgery, ask that doctor, as well as your primary care physician, the following questions.

- Are there alternatives? What are the consequences of not having the surgery? (If you are still in doubt, get a second opinion from a physician not affiliated with the physician who recommended the operation.)

- What risk is involved? Feel free to ask questions. Even the most minor forms of surgery have some degree of risk, and you have the right to have that spelled out in advance. If you want an explanation of tests and other procedures to expect, ask for it. Unanswered questions can produce anxiety.

- Can you be under the care of your primary care physician or a hospital physician who specializes in diabetes?

WHEN TO GET A SECOND OPINION

You may want to get a second opinion when a doctor recommends surgery, long-term medication, or other treatments that will drastically affect your lifestyle. You may also want a second opinion when your doctor says there is no known therapy or calls the problem incurable. Some insurance companies insist on a second opinion before they pay full coverage for certain treatments. Others will pay some reimbursement for the second opinion.

Check with your insurance company to determine whether the medical costs for the recommended procedure are covered. Also, ask your insurance company whether they cover the cost of a second opinion. Ask, too, whether they pay only if you see one of the consultants they recommend.

Who to Ask

When you are searching for a physician to provide a second opinion, first ask your physician or other doctor you trust. Look for a doctor who is board certified in the field in which you are seeking information, such as cardiology or surgery. Be sure to tell the physician about your diabetes.

If the problem is diabetes related, call your local chapter of the ADA for names of specialists in your area.

(Cont.)

(Cont.)

For non-diabetes-related problems, try calling the appropriate department of a major medical center or teaching hospital. Ask for the name of a specialist in the field.

What to Ask

■ What is the diagnosis, and how was it determined?

■ What treatments are available, and which are most used?

■ Why do you suggest this particular treatment for me?

■ What is the success rate of the treatment?

■ Is the treatment reversible?

■ What are the potential side effects and complications of the treatment, and how likely are they?

■ Is the problem or the treatment likely to affect my diabetes control?

■ How long will I have to be in the hospital or undergo treatment? Will I need follow-up care?

■ Are there hidden costs associated with this treatment, such as repeated blood tests, physical therapy, or postoperative skilled nursing care?

■ Is this an experimental treatment? Will I be participating in research? If so, you'll need to evaluate the potential side effects and make sure that they do not outweigh the benefits.

If time allows, work with your physician to bring your diabetes under reasonably good control before you are hospitalized. This will improve your general health, which can help you withstand the stresses of surgery and may help reduce the chances of infections and speed healing after the operation. If your diabetes is poorly controlled when you enter the hospital, don't panic. Often a condition requiring emergency surgery will cause blood glucose levels to skyrocket. The hospital physicians and staff should be able to bring your blood glucose level into an acceptable range for the surgery. A carefully monitored insulin drip during surgery may be the correct treatment for you, especially if you normally rely on insulin injections. Ask your primary care physician to be by your side as much as possible. It's important for your surgeon and your physician to agree on all treatment.

Here's a preview of what to expect if you are scheduled for surgery. The surgeon will meet with you at least once before your operation to explain the surgery and what to expect afterward. It's a good idea to have a list of questions ready for when your surgeon comes by. The anesthetist (the health-care professional who administers anesthesia to keep the surgery painless) will visit you before surgery to tell you what to expect and, sometimes, to explain your alternatives. Nurses caring for you will also be able to answer many of your questions and concerns.

After the operation, do not hesitate to ask for medication for pain or nausea if you are uncomfortable. Short-term use of these medications does not interfere with blood glucose control.

Blood Glucose Level in the Hospital

If your usual routine for controlling your blood glucose is working well when you enter the hospital, your physician will probably not want to tamper with it. But expect the hospital staff to keep close tabs on your blood glucose levels. The stress caused by the impending surgery, the condition making the surgery necessary, and the changes in your eating and exercise habits may upset control, especially toward the day of surgery.

If that happens, and if you usually control your diabetes with diet alone or diet plus an oral medication, don't be alarmed if the physician decides to put you on insulin. It's almost always a temporary measure, and once the stresses of hospitalization are over, you should be able to resume your usual routine.

Typically, for temporary insulin users, the doctor will prescribe insulin to be injected several times a day. The number of injections and dosages of the insulin will be adjusted based on the results of blood glucose tests. For these tests, glucose is usually measured at the bedside with the same kind of meter you may be using.

Some physicians may prefer to give you insulin continuously, directly into a vein (intravenously, or IV). At the same time you will probably also receive glucose intravenously. By

47

adjusting the flow of insulin and glucose and checking your blood glucose frequently, those attending to you should be able to keep your blood glucose level stable.

Don't expect your blood glucose levels to be in the same range as they were before entering the hospital. Your physician may want to keep them higher than normal, to avoid the possibility of a hypoglycemic reaction. Most physicians agree that having blood glucose levels slightly higher than normal (but under 200 mg/dl) for a few days is unlikely to do you any long-term harm. But if you feel symptoms of high or low blood glucose levels, don't hesitate to tell a doctor or nurse and ask for a blood glucose test.

For some operations, you may be able to eat by that evening or the next morning. For others, you may not be able to eat for several days and may require IV feeding, including glucose. If this is your case, your blood glucose level should be checked frequently.

BRINGING CARE HOME: HOME HEALTH CARE

You may find yourself turning to home health care in a variety of situations. Home health care can include medical professionals who help you when you're bedridden with a long illness or housebound for a short period. Services provided by home health-care agencies include nursing care and physical, respiratory, occupational, or speech therapy; chemotherapy; nutritional guidance; personal care such as bathing and dressing; and homemaker care. They may provide blood testing or bring a nurse into your home to administer drugs and other treatments. Home health-care workers include professionals, paraprofessionals (a trained aide who assists a professional), and volunteers.

Check your health insurance plan or ask your company benefits officer about coverage for home health care. Don't hesitate to ask the home health-care agency you are considering hiring how much they charge for each service. Ask your insurance company which of these charges will be covered. If you are covered by Medicare, some limited home health-care coverage may be available to you. These benefits apply only to those 65 or older or to those under 65 who need kidney dialysis and/or transplants. Medicare also covers the seriously disabled who have received Social Security disability payments for a two-year period. Usually Medicare home health-care benefits are restricted to the homebound and bedridden. (Ask the home health-care agency whether they have met Medicare standards.)

Veterans Affairs, the military, and worker's compensation can be other sources of financial help for home health care. To find out more about home health care, see Resources.

NURSING HOME OPTIONS

If full-time care is needed, a nursing home is often the best option. If you are researching nursing homes, some good sources of help include:

- A private or public case management social workers
- Your local office on aging

FRINGE BENEFITS OF DIABETES

When I was diagnosed as having diabetes several years ago, the first thing I did was read everything I could find on my newly acquired chronic disease. The picture painted was not exactly upbeat. One writer capsulized the general outlook by saying there would never be a book titled *The Joy of Diabetes*. Maybe not, but it did not take me long to discover that, despite the pessimistic literature on the subject, my disease was not without its benefits.

For example, when approached by teeming hordes of children selling candy to raise money for their school, I no longer have to make excuses about not being able to find my wallet. Now I just say, I am sorry but I have diabetes, at which time most children leave meekly, even the ones who don't know really what diabetes is.

Perhaps the biggest advantage of diabetes is that it makes you appreciate what you've got. I know I'm never going to experience an existential crisis. Even if I should ever make enough money to satisfy my every material desire, I'll never take life for granted. The disease itself gives your life a purpose—to try to maintain your health so you can enjoy what the future brings.

—*Robert A. Fellman, Nashville, Tennessee*

- The county or state department of health
- Your primary care physician
- Your religious leader or pastoral counselor
- Local organizations for the retired or elderly.

You will want to visit prospective sites. It's also a good idea to talk with friends, neighbors, or coworkers who have family members in nursing homes.

Nursing homes can be very expensive. There are four possible sources of payment: private insurance, Medicare, Medicaid, and self-pay or private pay. Different facilities ask for different types of payments. It's important to clarify what you get for the fees paid. The admissions coordinator should provide details of regular monthly charges and exactly what they do—and do not—include. Ask specifically whether there is something you should know about that is not covered.

To get more information about selecting and paying for a nursing home, see Resources.

Living Every Day With Type II Diabetes

After you discovered you had diabetes, members of your health-care team probably suggested a treatment routine consisting of goals for meals, exercise, and medication (if necessary). Hopefully, you then spent some time figuring out ways to care for yourself as an individual. If not, start now! Trial and error is the only way to find what works best for you. Schedules and meal and exercise plans are an important part of each day. It is up to you to try out these treatment plans and, after discussion with your health-care team, make adjustments that make them a realistic part of your life.

How do you know whether your treatment plan is working? This is where monitoring comes in. "Monitoring" may sound technical, but it's really just a way of assessing how well you are managing your diabetes. Instead of simply saying to yourself, "I feel fine," or "I feel lousy," you take measurements and keep records. For example, measuring how much you weigh is a simple yet important kind of monitoring you need to do.

Monitoring your blood glucose levels will primarily be your responsibility. Other ways of monitoring your health, such as blood cholesterol levels and kidney function, will be done by your primary care physician. Monitoring your blood pressure may be done by both you and your health-care team. Each of these ways of monitoring your health will provide the information you and your health-care team need to create the most effective plan for living the life you want with diabetes.

MONITORING THAT YOU CAN DO

Blood Glucose

Compared with people with type I diabetes, blood glucose levels in type II diabetes tend to show less variation throughout each day and from day to day. If your diabetes is successfully controlled by diet and exercise only, you may feel that you do not need to perform self-monitoring of blood glucose (SMBG), unless you become ill. However, learning to perform SMBG provides you with a valuable tool for understanding the impact of diet (and individual foods), exercise, and stress on your blood glucose level. Testing your blood gives you a record of how well you're handling your health and can motivate you to make improvements.

If your diabetes control regimen consists of diet and exercise plus oral medication, you may need to perform SMBG, at least until you and your health-care team are familiar and satisfied with your response to the drug and dosage you're taking. Determining the correct dose of oral medication can be as tricky as finding the right amount and time of insulin injections in individuals who require them. You could be surprised by unexpected bouts of hypoglycemia. The recommended times for SMBG are before breakfast and either before dinner or before going to sleep at night; occasionally, you may need to test two hours after breakfast and dinner.

You should test frequently on sick days, when your blood glucose levels are too high, when there are changes in your meal or exercise plans, when traveling, or when you suspect you are beginning to have a hypoglycemic reaction. If you typically have high blood glucose levels in the morning, check to see whether this is a result of "rebounding" from a very low blood glucose level while you sleep. Perform SMBG around 3:00 AM, and if you discover hypoglycemia, treat it as you normally would. Be sure to tell your primary care physician about your findings.

As you lose weight, so that the reduction in insulin resistance once again balances your ability to secrete insulin, you may that find your dose of oral medication is too strong. One sign of this is frequent bouts of hypoglycemia. Increase the number of times you check your blood glucose to three or four a day and whenever you feel like you are having hypoglycemia. Your records of SMBG will help both you and your primary care physician in making the best decision about your treatment.

There are considerable differences in the timing and during of action of the various oral diabetes medications. In addition, individuals differ in the way their bodies use the medications. If you feel that your oral diabetes medication is not doing what it should be, your SMBG records will assist your primary care physician in deciding on a new course of treatment. Never change your dose on your own. You need advice from your health-care team.

At some point, your primary care physician may prescribe

insulin for you. Learning to inject insulin is easy for some people but hard for others. It means having to take a little more effort to care for yourself. Monitoring your blood glucose must be included in your insulin-injection routine. Depending on your insulin program, you may need to test several times each day. Ask your primary care physician when and how often you should perform SMBG.

Keeping records of the results of SMBG is important. You should keep all your results in one easy-to-use form. Ask your physician or diabetes educator for a record book. A few blood glucose meters have an extensive memory, which saves you from having to write your results down each time. Always show your records to each member of your health-care team.

Equip Yourself

Before you invest a lot of money in a blood glucose meter, talk with a diabetes educator about your needs and what equipment is available. Discuss with your primary care physician how often you should perform SMBG. There are aids for visually impaired people or people who have difficulty manipulating objects or holding objects steady. There are meters that "talk" or have a large results display designed for people who are visually impaired. Almost anyone can perform SMBG.

You may want to consider a meter with a memory or data-management system for storing each reading, along with information on meals, exercise, and medication dose. (Be sure your physician has the necessary office equipment to "download" your meter's memory and print out the accumulated information to review it with you.) However, writing down daily results in a record book allows you to familiarize yourself with the patterns of your blood glucose levels.

For occasional blood glucose readings, strips that indicate the glucose content in a drop of blood by a color change, which you then match visually to a color chart, will tell you your glucose reading fairly accurately. Your vision must be excellent to achieve good results with this method, although large color block comparison charts are available. There are aids for steadying your test strips for comparing them to the color chart. A much less accurate method is measuring glucose in a urine sample with a glucose-sensitive test strip just for this purpose. This method should be used as a last resort only. In many individuals, urine glucose levels have little relation to blood glucose levels. Not completely emptying your bladder each time can influence your results. Finally, the information you get is hours old—it's hard to act on past information.

Each fall, the American Diabetes Association's magazine for members, *Diabetes Forecast*, publishes a buyer's guide to diabetes products. Consider ordering a reprint of this section for

---

THE COLORS OF DIABETES

I never imagined my life would be tied to a strip of paper. Or that the colors brown, green, or blue could mean the difference between sickness and health.

Eight years ago, I was diagnosed with diabetes. The doctor put me on an 1800-calorie diet and oral medication. I was 34, so giving up sweets didn't seem like such a big deal.

I soon realized that sweets were the least of it. Try not eating when you're hungry. Try doing it the rest of your life—craving the next meal even before you've finished the one in front of you. Try explaining to your friends that you're on a diet when you just dropped 30 pounds and can't keep the weight on.

The little strips of paper kept turning up brown.

I tried to control my disease by diet, oral medication, and exercise. I became a nutrional information addict, studying the list of ingredients on every can and loaf of bread at the supermarket shelf, figuring out how I could eat the most food with the least carbohydrate kick. I'd get impatient when my wife would tell me I'd already eaten 2 Starch/Bread exchanges at dinner, how about a snack of raw vegetables instead? So I cheated.

And the little strips of paper kept turning up brown.

I bought a blue bicycle. On my lunch hour, I'd ride 15 miles in 50 minutes, burning off calories. It only made things worse. I'd be hungry all morning, eat my meager lunch, then bust my tail riding the bicycle—all to maintain a low blood glucose level. Afterward, I'd eat a couple of candy bars, telling myself I needed them. I'd earned them.

(Cont.)

(*Cont.*)

And the little strips of paper kept turning up brown.

Finally, I stopped glucose testing. I knew by now the strips would always turn up brown, proving I'd failed again.

Once a week or so, I'd take out a urine test strip and stare at it hard, fixing its blue color in my mind and praying it wouldn't change when exposed.

On New Year's Day five years ago, my wife drove me to the hospital emergency room. My blood glucose level was over 400. After four days in intensive care, I came back to the world. At first, I was too groggy to pay much attention to the insulin injections I was getting. Then, the nurses told me I'd have to learn to give myself shots before I could go home. Talk about instant motivation!

When I first learned I had diabetes, I told myself becoming insulin dependent would be like giving up my freedom. But I'm here to tell you that it's really just the opposite. With insulin therapy, I have the energy to carry on with my life, to be there for the people I love, and to ride my bicycle. Believe me, being insulin dependent can mean freedom.

And the little strips of paper keep turning up blue.

— *Terry Sanville, San Luis Obispo, California*

descriptions of the latest self-monitoring devices. Monitoring equipment changes from year to year. Try the mail-order supply companies that advertise in *Diabetes Forecast* when looking for the lowest prices for blood testing strips and other equipment.

How to Perform SMBG

Methods for blood glucose testing vary by manufacturer. Be sure to thoroughly understand the timing and technique for the product you choose. You should be instructed by a diabetes educator on how to perform SMBG. Your technique needs to be reviewed with a diabetes educator regularly, for example, during your physical exams. Illustrated SMBG method is given in the Appendix.

Dealing With Results

When learning how to do SMBG, you'll probably be concerned about performing the test correctly. If a reading you aren't expecting shows up, you might blame it on your technique or meter malfunction. (Always keep your meter calibrated according to the manufacturer's instructions.) As you become more confident, those concerns will disappear, but others will take their place.

If you are faced with an unexpected high or low blood glucose reading, you might be tempted to criticize yourself. Maybe you know why your blood glucose is higher than you would like—the extra helping you ate at dinner, or the pie you usually avoid. Record your blood glucose honestly, forgive yourself, and be glad you can figure out why it's high. It's really frustrating when it's high but you don't know why. A series of unexplainable high or low results should get you in contact with your primary care physician quickly.

You may feel you know what your blood glucose level is without testing by the way you feel. It's true that with a lot of training by specialists, you might be right somewhat more often than not. But that's not often enough—you may be someone who develops hypoglycemia suddenly and with very little warning. No studies have shown that anyone can predict their glucose level accurately all the time. So, test anyway— you might be surprised!

HANDLING EMERGENCIES

Dealing with high and low blood glucose levels are a fact of life with diabetes. Being prepared is your best bet, and frequent SMBG will prevent most emergencies. Learn to recognize the signs your body gives when your balance is off center. There is some evidence that people who have had diabetes for many years may be less aware of hypoglycemia. Rehearse your responses with your primary care physician and diabetes educator. Let a few trusted people around you know how to help you if you can't help yourself.

Watching Out for Hypoglycemia

If you inject insulin or take oral diabetes medications, there is a possibility that you could find yourself with more insulin available than your body needs—even if you always give yourself the same dose. How much insulin your body needs changes based on many things: how much food you eat, what kind of food you eat, how much exercise you get, when you exercise versus when you take your medication, the state of your health, how much stress you're under, and so on. It's almost impossible to control all of these things perfectly each day, even though you try. Insulin will do its job clearing the blood of glucose even if it means that glucose levels fall too low.

There are many signs of hypoglycemia; you need to pay attention to your own signs. They could be very different than what other people feel when their blood glucose dips too low. Watch out for shakiness, sweating, trouble concentrating, headache, dizziness, moodiness, clumsiness, tingling in your face, extreme hunger, or irritability. These symptoms can happen at any time—they can even wake you up in the night or cause you to have a nightmare. When you have a very low blood glucose level, you must treat it immediately.

Treating Yourself. If you think you are having hypoglycemia, you need to test your blood glucose level. Usually hypoglycemia means blood glucose levels less than 60 mg/dl, but ask your physician what levels **you** should be looking out for. If you cannot perform SMBG at that moment and you feel you are having hypoglycemia, the best thing to do is treat it immediately. Never wait until you get home, especially if you need to drive.

Treating your hypoglycemia does not mean eating treats! You might have a tendency to go overboard on sweet foods if you feel hypoglycemic, especially if you are on a weight-reducing diet. Use some restraint so you don't send your blood glucose levels soaring too much in the other direction. Here are some sample treatments for hypoglycemia:

- For quick, certain relief, 3 glucose tablets are best (available at the pharmacy)

- 2 tablespoons of raisins

- 1/2 can of regular soft drink

- 4 ounces of orange juice

- 4 ounces of skim milk

- 6 to 8 Lifesavers

Ask your primary care physician or dietitian for the treatment options that are right for you.

If your next meal or snack is more than 30 minutes away, have a follow-up snack after you have treated your hypoglycemia. Call your physician before your next dose of medication.

If you feel hypoglycemia occurring often, even with regularly scheduled meals and the usual amount of exercise, you need to perform SMBG and record your findings. Contact your primary care physician with your results to have your treatment adjusted promptly.

Severe Hypoglycemia. If symptoms of hypoglycemia go unnoticed or unheeded, you could develop severe hypoglycemia. When your blood glucose level is very low for a long time, your brain does not get enough glucose to maintain your consciousness, and you could become unconscious. This is a real emergency.

The best thing to do is avoid this situation by paying attention to your symptoms and treating yourself promptly. Also, be sure that family, close friends, and coworkers know the signs of impending severe hypoglycemia. If you are elderly and taking oral diabetes medications or insulin, you are at especially high risk for severe hypoglycemia.

Should you become unconscious, someone around you must take over. Calling for emergency help is the first step. Blood glucose level must be raised quickly. You will not be able to eat or drink anything; it could cause you to choke or drown.

The safest and most reliable remedy is to be injected with glucagon, a hormone secreted by the pancreas that quickly stimulates the liver to release glucose; it also inhibits insulin release. The injection technique is similar to injection of insulin. Someone you trust needs to be trained in how to fill the special glucagon syringe and inject you. Glucagon injection can cause vomiting, so the head needs to remain elevated above the stomach. Glucagon is available only as a prescription through your primary care physician. Although severe hypoglycemia is not common in type II diabetes, the sobering

59

news is that people taking long-acting oral diabetes medications still die of severe insulin reactions.

Controlling Hyperglycemia

People with type II diabetes generally do not have rapid or dramatic swings in their blood glucose levels compared with people with type I diabetes. But they can sustain higher than normal levels of blood glucose for long periods of time without symptoms or detection. This wears on the body and needs to be controlled. Chronic hyperglycemia is probably responsible for most of the accompanying health problems known as diabetes complications (see Chapter 5). Performing SMBG is the best way to gain control.

Acute Hyperglycemia. Life-threatening severe hyperglycemia can occur in people with type II diabetes. Blood glucose levels can soar over 600 mg/dl and even as high as 1,000 mg/dl. This sometimes happens when type II diabetes has yet to be discovered. Extreme hyperglycemia leads to dehydration. This is exactly what occurs in severe prolonged hyperglycemia, which can induce a coma.

Hyperglycemic hyperosmolar coma (HHC) is a condition that occurs almost exclusively in people with type II diabetes, especially those older than 50. Undiagnosed diabetes is responsible for HHC about a third of the time. Other people have just allowed their hyperglycemia to go uncontrolled for too long. HHC can be precipitated by stress, alcohol, untreated infection, or even a stroke. Sometimes deterioration in a person's ability to care properly for themselves (such not being able to get a glass of water due to loss of mobility), usually a result of age, contributes. Regular SMBG and visits to your primary care physician are the best steps you can take to prevent HHC.

MONITORING DONE BY YOUR HEALTH-CARE TEAM

You will visit your primary care physician several times a year. How often you need to visit depends on the state of your health. Most people with type II diabetes have two complete checkups a year—the works! You should expect your doctor to be thorough. How many other visits you make to your physician depends on how well you are doing. Intermediate visits may be scheduled every three to six months to check your blood pressure, eyes, and feet or to review your blood glucose levels. The more adjustments your medication needs, the more often you may need to be seen by your doctor.

It helps to be in good shape for complete checkups—no colds, well rested, and not unusually stressed out. On the other hand, your physician needs to see the real you. If there is something bothering you about your health, a checkup is the time to discuss it. It helps to start a list of your concerns and questions several weeks in advance of your appointment.

A Complete Physical Exam

A thorough physical exam will include, but not be limited to, the following aspects of your health.

- **Total body weight:** do you know the body weight that's best for you? Ask your doctor to tell you.

- **Blood pressure and pulse:** ask your doctor to tell you your blood pressure and pulse and your target levels.

- **Eyes:** although your eyes should be examined at least once a year by an eye doctor, including dilation of pupils, your primary care physician will check your eyes for easily observable problems and ask about any changes in your vision like loss of sharpness or seeing floating spots or flashes of light. The physician should look inside your eyes at the retina (the nervous tissue at the back of the eye that forms images) with an ophthalmoscope.

- **Heart:** this is most often done by listening to your heart through a stethoscope, although an electrocardiogram or even a stress electrocardiogram may be needed to detect symptom-free heart disease; these tests monitor the electrical activity and physical pumping of your heart muscle.

- **Feet:** with shoes and socks off (remove them yourself to remind your doctor to look each time you visit, not just during complete physicals), they will be checked for pulses, reflexes, calluses, infections, and sores.

- **Skin:** your largest organ will be examined by sight, with special attention to insulin-injection sites; point out any areas of concern, such as persistent dry or rough patches or changes you've noticed in moles or freckles.

- **Nervous system:** this will be examined by testing your reflexes and your ability to feel sharpness of a pin or the light touch of cotton or a brush. Bring up any persistent problems like dizziness on standing; pain, burning sensation, or numbness in your legs or arms; or constipation or diarrhea; difficulty urinating; or difficulty with erection or sexual satisfaction.

- **Mouth and neck:** this includes examining your gums, teeth, and mouth and throat tissues; feeling for swelling in the glands in your neck; and asking about your brushing and flossing habits. This does not replace visiting your dentist two or three times a year.

- **Blood:** a sample of blood will be used to examine the levels of glucose, glycosylated hemoglobin, fat (cholesterol and triglyceride), urea nitrogen, and serum creatinine (see below).

- **Urine:** examining a urine sample is one way your doctor has of determining how well your kidneys are working. If damage is occurring, the levels of protein or albumin, a specific type of protein, will be high. Later, they may lose the ability to filter the blood.

- **Asking questions:** your doctor should ask you to explain anything unusual you've noticed or any concerns you have.

More About Blood Pressure

Why is monitoring your blood pressure important? People with diabetes are twice as likely to develop high blood pressure (hypertension) than people without diabetes. Because it often lacks symptoms except in severe cases, high blood pressure can escape detection. If left undetected and uncontrolled, high blood pressure can worsen diabetes complications that involve blood vessels, such as eye disease (retinopathy) and kidney disease (nephropathy). (Read more about these complications in Chapter 5.) In the worst case scenario, a stroke or heart attack will be your first notice that you have high blood pressure. No one wants a surprise like that.

If you and your doctor are concerned about your blood pressure, it may be important to know your blood pressure in between office visits. Most hospitals will take it for you free of charge if you go to the emergency room and wait your turn. The blood pressure machines that take it for free in the pharmacy may or may not be accurate. You may decide you want to learn to take your own blood pressure.

It is easy to learn how to take your own blood pressure. The device you use, called a sphygmomanometer, can be purchased from a pharmacy without a prescription. Although the purchase will probably not be covered by your health insurance policy, the cost is modest, ranging from about $20 for a pump-up version with a stethoscope to around $50 for a digital readout model where no stethoscope is needed. Instructions are included with the sphygmomanometer, and the manufacturer usually gives a toll-free phone number if you have further questions about how to use it. Take it with you the next time you see your primary care physician so he or she can check your technique and the accuracy of your machine.

Normal or acceptable blood pressure readings differ between individuals, so ask your doctor to tell you your target blood pressure. Blood pressure is given as two numbers. The first number, systolic pressure, represents the force of your blood against blood vessel walls when your heart is pumping. The other number, diastolic pressure, tells this measurement when your heart is relaxed. Almost always, your physician will want to see a reading of less than 140 over 90.

Blood Testing

Glycosylated Hemoglobin. Your physician may call this test by another name: glycohemoglobin, hemoglobin A_{1c}, or just A_{1c}. Hemoglobin, the molecule contained in red blood cells that carries oxygen, adds glucose to itself when blood glucose levels are high. (All proteins in the body can combine with glucose when glucose levels are high. This glycosylation damages the protein, which may impair its ability to function properly.) Glucose stays on the red blood cell until it dies (red blood cell life span is about 120 days). Most tests measure the amount of glucose on just the A_{1c} kind of hemoglobin. The measurement is a percentage: a person without diabetes usually has less than 7 percent glycosylated hemoglobin; ask your physician what this number is with the test he or she uses. Your level should be close to 7 percent, too, if your diabetes is well controlled.

The reason the doctor measures glycosylated hemoglobin is because it gives a picture of your blood glucose levels over the past six to eight weeks. If your diabetes is stable, you will probably have this test two or three times a year.

Cholesterol and Other Blood Lipid Profiles. Do you know your cholesterol level? How about your level of triglycerides?

DIETARY FATS

When you read or hear something about dietary fats, the words saturated and unsaturated will always come up. Telling these kinds of fats apart can help you lower your blood fat levels. Here's why: saturated fats tend to contain cholesterol and also raise blood cholesterol levels; unsaturated fats usually contain little or no cholesterol and tend to lower blood cholesterol levels.

Foods usually contain a mixture of saturated and unsaturated fats. If the food you're questioning doesn't have a label to read (some labels don't break the fat into saturated versus unsaturated fat anyway), you can tell it contains mostly saturated fat if the fat in it is solid at room temperature. For example, saturated fat is found in foods from animals, such as butter, cream, meat fat, lard, cheese, and egg yolks.

Unsaturated fat is usually liquid at room temperature (and even in the refrigerator) and comes from vegetable sources, such as safflower or canola plants, and fish. The chemical difference between the two kinds of dietary fat is that unsaturated fat is missing one (monounsaturated) or more (polyunsaturated) pairs of hydrogen atoms. Adding the missing hydrogen atoms to vegetable oil to make it solid (called hydrogenation) turns unsaturated fat into saturated fat; examples are vegetable shortening and margarine.

Chances are good your primary care physician monitors these regularly. Keeping tabs on the levels of different fats in your blood is one way your primary care physician can monitor your risk of heart disease or circulatory problems.

Cholesterol is only one fatty material in your blood. The

other major kind of blood fat is called triglycerides. Cholesterol can be ingested in food from animal products or produced by the body; many cells have the ability to produce cholesterol— it's a necessary ingredient in body tissues. Other cells need to have cholesterol delivered to them. Triglyceride is the major kind of fat in foods. Triglycerides are also created by our bodies to store excess calories to provide energy at some future time. Neither of these kinds of fats can be dissolved in water (or the blood) and so must travel in the blood joined to proteins that carry them into and out of body tissues. These carrier proteins are called lipoproteins, merely a combination of the words lipid (fat) and protein.

The carrier proteins have been divided into three kinds by how big they are plus how much they weigh. Cholesterol carried by low-density lipoprotein, or LDL cholesterol, is the kind people talk about when they say "cholesterol"; LDL does most of the work carrying cholesterol in the blood. Excess levels of LDL cholesterol are deposited on artery walls, a condition called atherosclerosis (a kind of arteriosclerosis, or "hardening of the arteries"), and can obstruct the flow of blood through the artery—leading to stroke or heart attack.

Cholesterol carried by high-density lipoprotein, or HDL cholesterol, transports the cholesterol into the liver from the blood or artery wall, where it is used for other purposes. Because the removal of cholesterol from the blood and artery walls is beneficial, high levels of HDL cholesterol are considered to be important for good health

Problems with blood lipids are common in diabetes. They occur when blood glucose levels are abnormally high and when cholesterol and triglycerides eaten in foods or produced by the body exceed the body's needs. You might be surprised to learn that people with type II diabetes often have normal LDL cholesterol levels. Unfortunately, your high levels of triglycerides and/or low levels of HDL will be areas of concern instead.

Your primary care physician will probably check your levels of cholesterol and triglycerides once a year by taking a blood sample after a 12-hour fast. Total cholesterol level and levels of each type of cholesterol will be measured. If HDL cholesterol is high, rejoice! If LDL cholesterol or triglycerides are high, be prepared to improve your blood glucose control (if needed) and to start a diet low in saturated fats.

NORMAL* LEVELS OF BLOOD LIPIDS		
Total Cholesterol		
	Desirable	Under 200 mg/dl
	Borderline	200 - 240 mg/dl
	High	Over 240 mg/dl
LDL Cholesterol		
	Desirable	Under 130 mg/dl
	Borderline	130 - 159 mg/dl
	High	160 mg/dl or above
HDL Cholesterol		
	Low	Under 35 mg/dl
Triglycerides		
	Desirable	Under 200 mg/dl
	Borderline	200 - 399 mg/dl
	High	400 mg/dl or above

Like blood pressure, acceptable levels of blood lipids differ between individuals: ask your primary care physician to tell you your target levels. Men tend to have lower HDL and higher LDL cholesterol levels than women.

Testing Kidney Function

Protein. If the kidneys are damaged, they become less efficient at removing waste products from and returning important substances to the blood. Also, proteins and substances normally too large to escape from the blood into collecting tubules pass through leaks in the filtering system. A test for detecting very early kidney damage has become increasingly common. It can detect very small amounts of albumin, a type of protein that should not be lost, in the urine.

Urea Nitrogen and Creatinine. If your urine test showed that abnormal levels of protein are being lost from your body, your doctor will test your blood levels of urea nitrogen and creatinine. Instead of being returned to the blood by the kidneys, these two compounds should be removed from the blood. High levels of urea and creatinine in the blood indicate that there is a buildup of toxic compounds in the blood. Serious problems with kidney disease can occur in type II diabetes (especially when accompanied by hypertension) as in type I diabetes. High levels of any of these indicators would call for a diet low in protein and other measures. For more on kidney function, see Chapter 5.

YOUR EYE EXAMINATION

At least once a year, you need a complete eye examination. This should include dilation of your pupils with drops to check the health of the blood vessels that supply your retina.

Your primary care physician and eye-care professionals should work together to protect your vision. Your primary care physician should be alert to any problems that are presented during your examinations, with referral to an ophthalmologist if any symptoms like unexplained light flashes, objects floating across the visual field, or loss of sharpness are discovered or if hemorrhages or leakage of blood vessels are seen through the ophthalmoscope.

If, during the examination, your eye-care professional finds evidence of diabetic or high blood pressure blood vessel damage or a change in eye pressure, you should be referred to a retina specialist or ophthalmologist for treatment. Only retina specialists or ophthalmologists are qualified to perform the kinds of treatment that can stop further eye damage, such as laser therapy.

LOSING WEIGHT

If you have type II diabetes and are overweight, you have lots of company—more than 75 percent of all people with type II diabetes are, or were at one time, obese.

Obesity

What is obese? Medically, it means weighing more than 20 percent over your healthy body weight. For example, if your primary care physician tells you that your healthy weight is 150 pounds, adding any more than 30 pounds (weighing more than 180 pounds) qualifies you as obese.

What is a healthy weight for you? Your primary care physician or dietitian can tell you. In 1990, the U.S. Department of Health and Human Services for the first time issued two sets of suggested weight ranges for adults divided into those 19 to 34 years old and those 35 and older. It was finally recognized that people tend to gain weight after age 35 but that this weight gain will not necessarily lead to health problems. This flexibility will probably be echoed by your dietitian. Most dietitians are trained not only to look at weight/height charts but to help you define a weight goal based on personal and family history as well.

Fat

There's another aspect to what your healthy weight should be: how much of your weight is fat? Two adults who weigh the same can have very different states of health due to the difference in the amount of fat versus muscle they are carrying around. Although one pound of muscle equals one pound of fat on the scale, muscle works for its keep by burning calories. Fat, on the other hand, is stored energy, created when intake of food exceeds your body's energy needs for growth, repair, and activity.

Everyone needs to have some fat in their body. Women normally have more fat than men, an evolutionary tactic for having the energy reserves to deal with pregnancy and breastfeeding. Fat also serves as insulation and holds internal organs in their proper place. Most important, fat provides a source of energy for keeping us going between meals and during sustained physical activity.

Having too much body fat can be the result of eating too much and exercising too little. However, in some people, excess fat is a product of inherited disorders in fat metabolism (the way the body uses fat). There is much evidence that your genes have a lot to do with how much you weigh and how much fat you have. Although this makes it harder to do the "battle of the bulge," every effort should be made to reduce food intake appropriately and exercise more.

Extra food not used for body maintenance and physical activity is stored in fat cells as triglycerides. (Note that breaking down and using or storing ingested carbohydrates requires about eight times more energy, measured as calories burned, than storing ingested fat as triglycerides.) When blood levels of triglycerides are high, fat cells take up triglycerides until the fat cells are many times bigger than normal, and up goes insulin resistance. As the size, and sometimes the number, of your fat cells increases, up goes the amount of body fat. Adding to this is the fact that a lot of people who develop type

II diabetes already have unusually high blood levels of triglycerides.

Research has also found that the location of your body fat is related to your risk for specific diseases, diabetes and heart disease among them. Upper-body obesity (from the "belly" up), which is more common in men than women, appears to be caused by large, insulin-resistant fat cells that readily release the building blocks of fat, called fatty acids, into the blood. This type of body fat pattern is associated more with diabetes, hypertension, and heart disease than lower-body obesity (from the hips down), which is more common in women. Smaller fat cells that respond normally to insulin are responsible for lower-body obesity.

Fat and Insulin

How does being obese relate to diabetes? A general answer to this question is that having too much fat, particularly on the upper body, decreases your body's ability to use insulin. This is called insulin resistance.

Being overweight and overfat puts a strain on your pancreas to produce enough extra insulin to meet your needs. When this need isn't met, as time goes on, excess levels of glucose circulating in your blood eventually impair the efficiency with which the cells in your body take in and use glucose. This means even more glucose remains in your blood unused. So, blood insulin levels keep going up, but to no avail.

None of this happens overnight. It takes years, sometimes decades, of being overweight before chronic severe glucose intolerance, **diabetes**, occurs. You lessen your chances of developing type II diabetes dramatically by keeping yourself at your healthy body weight with a healthy body fat distribution. Once you have diabetes, achieving your healthy weight can mean freedom from medications or insulin injections. It can also bring years of good health and a smaller risk of diabetes complications.

A Loss You Can Live With

Motivating yourself to lose weight and fat may be your biggest challenge. Doing the right thing when you're faced with high-fat choices at a restaurant or at the snack machine is not easy. Filling the eating void is hard. It's best if you can fill the void with exercise, but this isn't always practical. Your challenge is to find the solution that works best for you. It is guaranteed, however, that you'll call on every ounce of patience you have.

MY MEAL PLAN

The first week, I measured my food. I balanced my categories. I was careful with exchanges. I didn't quite understand exchanges, but, book in hand, I'd try to figure it out. I talked to a dietitian and nodded agreement to all of her good plans. She worked out a sample menu, and I indicated understanding. I was faithful for a while, but this didn't seem to change the way I was feeling. I wasn't *really* sick.

Gradually, I began to estimate portions. I didn't feel any different. I was having trouble accepting the fact that I had diabetes and that these things were important. What harm would it do to have one cookie? Nothing happened—why not have two? Have ice cream for a special treat? Sure!

The special treat happened more and more frequently. The holidays came, and I felt deprived. Why limit myself? I'm not *really* sick, and I don't need to watch what I eat. I needed comfort and used food for comfort. I kept saying, "I'll begin again tomorrow." When tomorrow came, I would begin again and fail. I'd start again and again and fail again and again.

—*Mary J. Eno, Melrose, Massachusetts*

No one plan for losing weight works for everyone. Your best bet is to get some people to cheer you on: your dietitian, your primary care physician, and your family and friends. Your dietitian will discuss acceptable approaches to weight loss with you, such as

- Nutritionally sound, modestly calorie-restricted low-fat meal plans that achieve slow, gradual weight loss over several months

- Increased physical activity

- Behavior modification through a goal and reward system

■ In special circumstances and under close supervision by your primary care physician, a nutritionally balanced very-low-calorie diet (for 3 months or less).

Perhaps the most important advice is this: set realistic goals. Do not try to lose weight too fast. A steady loss of 1 pound a week is a safe and effective means to reach your goal. You probably know someone who lost a lot of weight quickly only to gain it back. (Research is providing evidence that such swings in body weight may pose other health hazards.) Go for long-term success by developing better eating and exercise habits. Set short-term goals, for the day or the week, and take it one day at a time. Chapter 4 discusses creating a healthy individualized meal plan.

THE VALUE OF EXERCISE

You probably already know that exercise is good for you. It is especially good for people with diabetes because it lowers blood glucose levels and improves the flow of blood through the small blood vessels. It improves the heart's pumping power. It helps you control stress. Adding regular exercise to your diet program will speed up your weight loss. The other major benefit is that regular exercise may improve the way insulin works in your body. There's a good chance that successful diet therapy plus exercise can alone control your diabetes. What other chronic disease can be treated so successfully just by maintaining good habits?

Exercise appears to improve blood glucose control especially effectively in people with type II diabetes. One explanation for improved blood glucose control is that exercise affects the ability of muscles to take in and use glucose not only during exercise but also for hours afterward. (People with type I diabetes find this out when they have unexpected hypoglycemia hours after they've finished exercising.)

Your muscles use glucose for energy during periods of sustained work. A short burst of activity would probably be fueled by glycogen, the stored form of glucose. However, as activity continues, after you are "warmed up," stored glycogen is used up, and the cell will pull more and more glucose from a ready source: your blood. The activities within the cell that allow it to use glucose are speeded up. Little or no insulin is required for this kind of glucose use.

Even after muscle contraction stops, your muscle cells stay busy gathering more glucose to replenish glycogen stores. People who exercise find that their muscles burn more fuel even when they aren't exercising. You might think of this as an increase in your metabolism.

If you still need more incentive to start and stick to an exercise program, how about this: a long-term exercise program can prevent heart disease, lower triglyceride and cholesterol levels, improve mild hypertension, and improve your outlook on life. People have reported an increased sex drive when on an exercise program. Exercise is not a cure-all, but it's close!

Creating a Lifestyle That Includes Exercise

You should see your primary care physician before you begin any new exercises or exercise program. Your doctor or an exercise specialist will be able to advise you about or design a program especially for you. If you have special considerations— neuropathy or loss of feeling, obesity, pregnancy, loss of mobility—don't worry. There are exercise plans for you. Your first step could be as simple as a walk every night after dinner or taking the stairs instead of the elevator.

How happy you are fitting exercise into your life will determine your success. Finding activities that you enjoy will enhance your desire to do them. Remember, half the battle is showing up. Once you force yourself to get into the workout clothes and arrive at class or get into the pool, you'll be glad you did. And you'll have something to be proud of—your behavior. Stick with it! Within three months, about the time it takes most people to form a new habit, you'll wonder how you ever got along without exercise.

DIABETES MEDICATIONS

Diet therapy, weight loss, and regular exercise are the best treatments for type II diabetes. However, if you are newly diagnosed with type II diabetes and have high blood glucose levels or if your success on these treatments has been limited, your doctor may prescribe medication. Medications that lower blood glucose levels come in two forms: oral medications and insulin injections. Both can be prescribed in the treatment of type II diabetes. Taking a pill or injecting insulin, however, will not make your type II diabetes go away. Look at it as an aid to getting your blood glucose control on the right track.

Oral Medications

Discovered by accident in the 1940s, sulfonylurea drugs lower blood glucose by encouraging the pancreas to produce and release more insulin, decreasing the release of glucose by the liver, and overcoming insulin resistance by the muscles. No one is sure exactly how all this happens. Five different sulfonylureas are commonly prescribed in the U.S.: tolbutamide (brand name Orinase), Tolazamide (Tolinase), glyburide (Diabeta or Micronase), glipizide (Glucotrol), and chlorpropamide (Diabinase). Glyburide and glipizide are the most recent additions to the group and are termed "second generation" oral agents. Drugs of the second generation work effectively in smaller doses than those of the first generation.

Sulfonylureas are not the only oral hypoglycemic medications. Drugs called biguanides are prescribed frequently in Europe to people with type II diabetes. However, the use of biguanides for treating type II diabetes was banned in the U.S. in the 1970s because the one in use was too often associated with side effects. A safer biguanide called metformin is being investigated for use in the U.S.

Your doctor will consider your lifestyle, physical condition, and needs before prescribing a particular sulfonylurea drug to you. For instance, tolbutamide may be the safest sulfonylurea drug for an older person living alone, because it has a minimal risk of hypoglycemia. On the other hand, the effects of chlorpropamide can continue an unexpectedly long time—up to and beyond 36 hours.

Oral medications come in tablet form. You will be responsible for taking the medication once or twice a day. As with any prescription, you should be certain how your doctor wants you to take this drug before you leave the office. "How much?" and "When?" are two questions you need to have your doctor answer.

Interactions and Side Effects. It is especially important for you and your doctor to discuss every other medication, prescription or over-the-counter, that you are currently taking

73

or might be thinking about taking. These can include aspirin, thyroid or high blood pressure medicine, medicine to lower blood cholesterol, and cold and allergy medicines. Drugs can interact with each other to cause sickness or ill health that might be difficult to diagnose. Some drugs can have the side effect of lowering or increasing blood glucose; their effects must be taken into consideration so that your blood glucose level doesn't go too low or stay too high. The symptoms of drug interactions can be mistaken for hypoglycemia and mistreated. Many drugs interfere with the body's use and elimination of oral diabetes medications and may indirectly cause hyper- or hypoglycemia.

Taking any sulfonylurea drug increases your risk for severe hypoglycemia, especially if you skip meals or drink too much alcohol. Be sure to discuss with your doctor what symptoms to watch for and let your family and other people you see often know what these symptoms look like. Formulate an action plan with your doctor for how to deal with hypoglycemia caused by your oral agent.

Besides hypoglycemia, other side effects can include an interaction with alcohol that makes you feel flushed or nauseated and have a rapid heartbeat (especially with chlorpropamide). In rare instances, your body may retain water, causing headache, sleepiness, nausea, or convulsions, or you may develop skin irritations and rashes. Tell your doctor about any changes you notice in your behavior or body after you begin treatment with a sulfonylurea drug or after a change in dosage.

Who Benefits From Oral Medications? Not all people with type II diabetes respond to treatment with oral medications. People likely to show lowered blood glucose levels are those who have had hyperglycemia for less than 10 years, who are normal weight or obese (the pills work poorly in very thin people), who are willing to follow a healthy meal plan, and who have some insulin secretion by their pancreas.

You should not take sulfonylurea drugs if your pancreas no longer secretes insulin (as in type I diabetes) or if you are pregnant, have allergies to sulfa drugs, or have significant liver or kidney disease. During severe infections or major surgery, oral diabetes medications may have to be replaced or supplemented with insulin injections temporarily.

Before prescribing oral drugs, your doctor should first put you on diet and exercise therapy. You must continue managing your diet and getting enough exercise if you later have to start taking oral medication. The best effects are achieved through a total effort.

LIFE SINCE DIAGNOSIS

After my diabetes diagnosis, I spent the next 10 days in the hospital and began both insulin injections and a patient/family education program. My wife was very relieved to learn that diabetes was a condition we could deal with successfully. I was released and told to take insulin daily. Looking back now, I suppose it was a sort of forced New Year's resolution to take care of myself.

The next 15 months were filled with fear, anxiety, and adjustment for my family and me, but it was all worth it. I had to eat six small meals a day at regular times. Meals became a family project, and we all have better eating habits now. Instead of eating large amounts of fried, salty, and sweetened foods, we eat fish, poultry, fresh salads, and lots of fruits and vegetables.

By March 1985, I had lost a total of 60 pounds and gradually reduced my insulin dose. I felt better than I had in the past six years!

During that month an unexpected and wonderful thing happened. All the dieting and exercise paid off when my doctor suggested I go without insulin for a few days. I haven't taken insulin or diabetes medication in any form since then, and I'm feeling great!

My blood glucose levels are under control, my life is back to normal. But now the rules are stricter. Attention to my diet and regular exercise are a must.

Life since diagnosis has not been problem free. But at 56, I have learned to listen to my body and know how to handle diabetes.

—*Carl M. Ward, Harrisonburg, Virginia*

After you have had consistently normal fasting blood glucose levels (115 to 140 mg/dl) for several weeks or months, it's possible that you can control your hyperglycemia by diet and exercise alone. Ask your doctor to put you on a trial of diabetes control with no pills, just diet and exercise. But continue to self-monitor your blood glucose!

There is the possibility that sulfonylurea treatment won't help you or that it will help you, but just for a while. In people who have initial success with oral diabetes medications, about 5 to 10 percent stop responding within a year; another 50 percent eventually stop responding. In people who have some characteristics of type I diabetes when diagnosed with type II diabetes, oral diabetes medications usually stop helping their hyperglycemia within two years. If oral treatment fails, your doctor may then choose to add insulin to your treatment routine, with or without sulfonylurea therapy as well. If this seems the best course of treatment, you'll need to pay special attention to instructions and medication techniques and times. With this treatment will come a risk of hypoglycemia until your doctor finds the right doses for you. Write instructions down and spend time with a diabetes educator until you feel comfortable with your new treatment. Know your symptoms of hypoglycemia, treat it immediately, and call your physician before your next dose of medication.

Insulin Therapy

Insulin must be injected into the body. Other ways of getting it into the body, such as by taking pills, have not proved successful yet.

Insulin as a treatment for type I diabetes began in the 1920s. The results were dramatic. Insulin and high-calorie diets were used to treat the high blood glucose levels of young people with type I diabetes instead of starvation diets, turning them from skeletons into chubby, healthy children within months.

The two main kinds of insulin are pork and human. Pork insulin is made by removing and purifying insulin from pig pancreases. Human insulin, however, is made in laboratories by inserting the human gene into bacteria or yeast and purifying the insulin that is made by these organisms. Most people who need insulin are started on human insulin because it is thought that there is less chance that the body will recognize it as "foreign." However, pork insulin is just as effective in lowering blood glucose levels. Your physician can advise whether you need to switch if you are taking one of the other insulins. Serious allergic reactions to any insulin are rare.

Your doctor will consider which kind of insulin is best for you. There are many choices by brand name and time of action. Insulins are divided into categories by how long they can act in the body after being injected. Short-acting (Regular) insulins go to work within 30 minutes and are used up in 6 to 8 hours. The effects of animal-source long-acting (Ultralente) insulins build slowly and last a long time—up to 48 hours. Human Ultralente lasts up to 24 hours. Intermediate (NPH or Lente) insulins fall somewhere in between (16–24 hours). Different doses and combinations of insulins can be prescribed and mixed in one syringe by you. There is even a premixed combination of 70 percent intermediate-acting and 30 percent short-acting insulins. Premixed insulins are especially helpful for those with dexterity or eyesight problems that can make drawing different amounts of insulin from two different bottles difficult. However, factors such as place of injection, insulin temperature, and whether your body has formed insulin antibodies may delay or accelerate insulin action. Insulin comes in one strength, called U-100 (100 units per cc).

Before you leave your doctor's office, be sure you understand what kind of insulin you are going to be taking, where you should inject it, what mixtures (if any) you need to prepare, how often to give yourself injections, and when to give them. Be clear about the relationship of your insulin injection and your meal times. Go step by step through a typical day, and talk about how to adjust for an unusual day—oversleeping, sickness, or travel.

Injecting Insulin. You will be more confident about starting insulin injections if you assemble the right equipment. When you pick up your insulin prescription, you'll need to buy syringes, also by prescription. You may have to try several brands of syringes before you find one that suits you.

- Your syringe should be designed to hold U-100 insulin.

- The syringe should be large enough to hold your entire dose for each injection; for example, if you take 45 units total dose, you cannot use a 30-unit syringe.

- Can you read the markings on the syringe easily? Would it help if the plunger were a different color?

77

■ You'll want the most comfortable syringe you can find. Disposable syringes with lubricated microfine needles will give you the smoothest penetration of your skin and will be the least painful. Ask your doctor or pharmacist to help you find the most comfortable needles.

Insulin stored long term needs to be kept cool but not frozen. However, injecting cold insulin can be uncomfortable. It is okay to keep the bottle of insulin you use every day at room temperature (use this rule of thumb: if you are comfortable, your insulin is, too). Ask your pharmacist or doctor to tell you proper ways of storing insulin. For special storage guidelines for insulin mixtures, see the Appendix. Also, insulin can "spoil." If you see any clumping or crystallizing in your insulin bottle, don't use it.

Make sure that you have learned the proper techniques for filling your syringe with insulin and for injecting yourself. Your doctor or diabetes educator should go over your technique with you until you feel confident about doing it on your own. The basic steps to preparing a syringe for injection are given in the Appendix.

Insulin-Injection Aids. If you have difficulty with any part of your insulin-injection routine, discuss your particular problem with your physician or diabetes educator. There are alternatives to traditional insulin delivery by syringe, and there are aids to help if vision impairment or loss of dexterity or steadiness is causing your difficulties.

You may want to consider a spring-loaded metal syringe if you are having problems manipulating the needle and syringe plunger. If you would like something other than a syringe, there are infusers, insulin pens, and jet injectors. Infusers are needles that remain taped in place at the injection site for two to three days. Insulin is injected into this needle rather than injecting through the skin in a new place each time. There is a risk of infection with this aid.

Insulin pens are filled like cartridge ink pens. Instead of ink, the cartridges are purchased prefilled with insulin. Only a few types of insulin are available in cartridges. You can set a dial on the pen that controls the amount of insulin released from the cartridge during the injection. Insulin pens are convenient for people who take multiple doses each day.

Jet injectors use pressure to move insulin across the fatty tissue instead of a needle. Although this may be the method for you, injectors are expensive, and there are sometimes problems with bruising or tearing of the skin or faster-than-desired insulin absorption.

If your vision is making insulin injection difficult, ask your health-care team about products that can assist you. There are syringe magnifiers that enlarge the markings on the syringe barrel, dose gauges that help you measure an accurate insulin dose (even mixed doses), and needle guides and vial stabilizers that help you insert your needle into the insulin vial to draw up your dose.

Choosing Your Injection Site. The areas chosen most commonly for insulin injection have a layer of fat under the skin above the muscle. The abdomen, except for a two-inch circle around the navel, is the most commonly used site and is often preferred because of better insulin absorption. Other areas are the top of the thighs when you're sitting, the backs of the

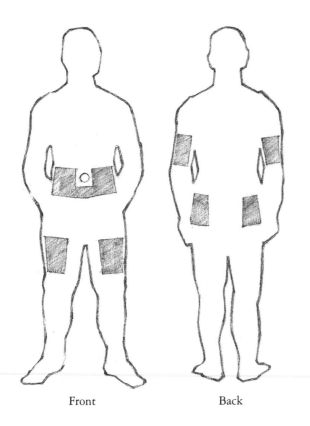

Front   Back

upper arms, the hips, and the buttocks. Discuss with your doctor or diabetes educator which areas are right for you.

Another important topic to discuss with your doctor or diabetes educator is how you should vary your injection site. Repeated injections in the same place can cause swelling, lumping, or indentation in the skin. These are changes in the fat layer under your skin. Varying your injection site or using different places within the same body area lets your fatty tissue recover from the injection and cuts down on your chances of developing scar tissue. Until you establish a daily routine, it's a good idea to keep a chart showing where you injected your insulin each time you do it.

The absorption of insulin is slower or faster depending on where it is injected. Here are some things to consider.

- In general, the abdomen absorbs insulin best, followed by the arms, thighs, and buttocks.

- Exercising a body part that has just received an insulin injection can speed the insulin absorption unpredictably. It is a good idea to avoid this problem. If you are just about to exercise your legs, for example by walking or riding your bike, don't inject insulin into your thigh. Use a site less likely to be directly involved in the exercise.

Syringe Reuse. The decision about whether to use your syringe more than once is up to you. There is no evidence that reusing a properly maintained syringe leads to increased rates of infection. However, if you have poor personal hygiene, are ill, have open wounds on your hands, or have decreased resistance to infection for any reason, you should not risk syringe reuse. Talk to your diabetes educator when you are deciding whether to reuse your syringes.

There are several reasons to consider reusing your syringes. You can save yourself money. You can save yourself the trouble of keeping up large supplies of syringes. Every syringe you reuse means a little less nondegradable plastic littering the earth. Before plastic syringes, people routinely boiled and reused glass syringes.

The American Diabetes Association offers guidelines if you choose to reuse your syringes (see the Appendix). Manufacturers of disposable syringes recommend that they be used only once because the sterility of a reused syringe cannot be guaranteed.

The most important advice about syringes is this: never let anyone use a syringe you've already used, and don't use anyone else's syringe, ever.

Syringe Disposal. When a syringe has finished being useful to you, make sure you do the right thing with it. Proper disposal of medical waste such as used syringes is important to everyone, from your trash collector to the members of your household to people using beaches and other public areas—in other words, how you do it affects everyone who can have contact with your trash.

Clipping the needles off the syringes is the best first step, but only if you do it correctly. Removing the needle will prevent anyone from ever using the syringe again. It's best to buy a device that clips, catches, and contains the needle. Do not use scissors to clip off needles—the flying needle could hurt someone or become lost. If you don't destroy your needles, recap them if you can do it safely. Place the needle or entire syringe in an opaque (not clear) **heavy-duty** plastic or metal container with a screw cap or other closing method. You don't want the syringes to escape once you've sent them to the dump. Do not use a container that will allow a needle to break through and possibly give someone an accidental needlestick— and lots of worry!

Note that your area may have special regulations for disposing of medical waste. Ask your refuse company or city or county waste authority whether the disposal method explained above meets their requirements. When traveling, bring your used syringes home; pack them in a heavy-duty container, such as a hard plastic pencil box, for transport.

81

Healthy Habits: Taking Care of Your Diabetes

CHAPTER 4

YOUR HEALTHY EATING PLAN

Chances are, there is nothing you can do that will help you live better with diabetes than changing your eating habits. As you develop healthy food strategies, you'll be examining what you eat, how you eat, and even when you eat. This is difficult work. Don't think you have to face it alone. As with any aspect of living well with diabetes, your health-care team can help.

Your goal in living well with diabetes has two parts:

- Keeping your blood glucose levels in the normal range.

- Avoiding short-term (low or high blood glucose reactions) and decreasing your risk of long-term complications of diabetes.

Diet is such an important way to care for yourself, the American Diabetes Association has almost 50 publications devoted to the subject. However, having diabetes doesn't change the facts of good nutrition. Healthy food choices for you are basically the same as healthy food choices for anyone else. In fact, your entire family can benefit from the food choices, cooking techniques, and meal planning that you learn.

Losing weight, if you need to, is often the most effective therapy for type II diabetes. For some people, even a modest weight loss, for example 5 to 15 pounds, can bring a dramatic improvement in glucose levels. A nutrition plan may help with hypertension or unhealthy lipid levels, too—both of which can contribute to the development of diabetic complications.

Nutrition Basics

Most of the calories in the food you eat are changed into glucose during digestion and as they're used (metabolized). In diabetes, your body has trouble metabolizing its fuel (food) properly. The result is that high levels of glucose are circulating in your blood. Avoiding any foods that would raise your blood glucose level is impossible.

Often, obesity accompanied by insulin resistance precedes type II diabetes. You may have other health problems in addition to diabetes, such as high blood pressure or high levels of blood lipids (triglycerides).

Good nutrition for anyone involves eating a variety of foods. This is because no one food can supply all the nutrients your body needs to stay healthy and active. Variety also keeps your meals from becoming boring. The main nutrients in food are carbohydrates, proteins, fats, vitamins, and minerals.

Carbohydrates give you energy. Carbohydrates come in two forms—simple and complex. **Simple carbohydrates** or sugars and refined flours—cakes, pastries, soft drinks, and candy, for example—tend to raise blood glucose to high levels quickly and provide few, if any, essential nutrients and no fiber. **Complex carbohydrates**—vegetables, dried beans and peas, brown rice, and whole-grain flours, breads, and cereals, for example—tend to raise blood glucose levels more gradually over a longer period of time than simple carbohydrates. Complex carbohydrates contain a variety of vitamins and minerals as well as the most fiber per bite.

Fiber, the indigestible part of plants, is found in dried peas and beans, fruits, vegetables, and whole-grain cereals, and breads. Soluble fiber dissolves in water and forms a gel in the intestinal tract. This material slows down food absorption and is believed to help delay the absorption of ingested glucose into the blood. Soluble fiber is found in fruits, oatmeal, and dried beans and peas. Insoluble fiber doesn't dissolve in water, but retains water, swelling and moving substances along the intestinal tract with it. This kind of fiber helps with regular bowel movements. Insoluble fiber is found in wheat bran, vegetables, and whole grains. Fiber in foods needs to be chewed, and chewing is one of the pleasures of eating.

Unhealthy Foods

Good nutrition also means limiting fat and cholesterol from food. True, the body does require some dietary fat daily. But extra dietary fat is readily stored as body fat, whereas an equal number of calories derived from complex carbohydrates cannot be stored as fat as readily or easily. Fat is found in many foods. Red meat, dairy products (whole milk, cream, cheese, and ice cream), egg yolks, butter, salad dressings, vegetable oils, and many desserts are high in fat. To cut down on fat and cholesterol,

- Choose lean cuts of meat (look for descriptions like "loin" and "round"); remove visible fat. Eat more fish and poultry (without the skin). An ideal portion of lean meat, fish, or poultry is about the size of a deck of cards, or 3 ounces.

- Use diet margarine instead of butter; avoid using solid shortening.

- Drink low-fat (1% or 2%) or skim milk and eat low-fat or skim-milk cheeses.

- Limit the number of eggs you eat to four or less a week.

- Choose liver once a month or less.

Too much salt may worsen high blood pressure in some people. Many foods contain salt as sodium. Sometimes, you can taste it (as in pickles or bacon). But there is also "hidden" salt in many foods, such as cheeses, salad dressings, cold cuts, canned soups, and fast foods. Take the salt shaker off the table. When using salt or fat, remember: a little goes a long way.

Everyone should eat less sugar. Sugar consists of "empty" calories with no vitamins or minerals. Most of the foods around us contain more sugar than we know, especially fat-free baked goods. One 12-ounce can of regular soft drink has 9 teaspoons of sugar.

Moderate use of alcohol should be the rule. What's moderate? The U.S. Department of Health and Human Services defines moderate drinking as 1 drink per day for women and 2 drinks per day for men. One drink can be 1 12-ounce beer, 5 ounces of wine, or 1 1/2 ounces of 80-proof distilled spirits.

Taking the Lead

In the team approach to diabetes management, you are the crucial player. No where is this more true than in setting your nutrition goals. When it comes to meal planning, weight-loss strategies, and adopting new eating habits, you owe it to yourself to take an active role. The more involved you are, the more your nutrition action plan will reflect your needs, tastes, preferences, and lifestyle and the more likely you are to succeed.

As with all diabetes care, meal planning starts with a visit to your primary care physician. The other important team member when it comes to nutrition matters is your dietitian. If your physician is not currently working with a dietitian, ask about involving this health-care professional in planning your diabetes treatment. Chapter 2 includes a section on how to find and work with a registered dietitian.

Keep in mind that devising a workable meal plan takes time as well as some trial and error. You and your dietitian will be creating a flexible eating plan that will reflect—to the extent possible—your lifestyle, food preferences, and daily routine. It will be a plan tailored to help you meet your particular health goals: losing weight, improving blood glucose control, lowering your cholesterol count, or whatever other objectives you're striving for.

Just as developing a meal plan takes time, so does changing a lifetime of eating habits. Although you're ultimately aiming for a lifelong change, try to take it a day—or even a meal—at a time. Be patient, and give yourself enough time to be successful with your diet therapy.

There is no magic solution to changing your eating habits. For that matter, no superhuman willpower is required. Your most important resources are likely to be determination, dedication, and patience. Be involved. Help make choices. Speak up when something isn't working. Modify your plan with your dietitian's help. When you stumble, pick yourself up and try again. Help yourself by including

- **Instruction:** learn as much as you can about what you're doing and why

- **Encouragement:** whether it comes from a support group, family member, friend, or mental health counselor

- **Frequent follow-up and evaluation:** you and your dietitian and other relevant health-care team members should meet regularly to check your progress, acknowledge your success, and make changes as needed

- **Behavior modification therapy:** this can be an important aid to the tough task of changing such deep-seated and often complex behaviors such as eating habits

When you meet with your dietitian, decide how you answer these questions.

- What are my goals? Break them into long-range and short-term goals. For example, you may want to lose 25 pounds; set a smaller initial goal of losing 5 pounds in a month.

- How will my meal plan help me achieve my goals?

- How can I find reward in my meal plan? Which of my favorite foods can be included?

DIABETES THE ALASKAN WAY

Dan Kahklen, a full-blooded Thlinget Indian, is from the Raven Dog Salmon Clan of southeast Alaska. His wife, Sue, is half Thlinget, of the Eagle Wolf Clan. Dan, now 80, first learned he had diabetes 12 years ago. When he was diagnosed, his blood glucose level was over 400 mg/dl.

Back then, neither Sue nor Dan knew much about the disease or the importance of a nutritious diet. But today they are experts in choosing healthy foods. Their health clinic (Alaska Health Service clinic of the Southeast Alaska Regional Health Corporation) sent them to the Alaska Native Medical Center in Anchorage to learn about insulin and diet. Sue read heavily on the subject and even followed Dan's new food plan. Her reward: Dan's diabetes is under control, and she has dropped from 200 to 165 pounds.

"Because we are Alaska natives," Sue says, "we had to change our whole way of eating. We used to eat sweet rolls and doughnuts. We fried our foods and made jams and jellies with lots of sugar. We used to salt our fish heavily. That can't have been good for us. We ate a lot of fat, too."

Now Sue skins chicken and trims fat off meat before cooking. Both she and Dan use only natural fruits and fresh vegetables to sweeten their food, and they eat dietetic jam. Dan uses no butter or margarine.

Perhaps the biggest change is in the way they prepare fish. "I used to fry all our fish in an inch of oil," Sue says. "Now I spread a little oil onto a nonstick pan with a paper towel. I add a little bit of seasoned flour of my own, and nothing else."

They watch portions, too. "We used to eat one whole thick slice of king salmon per person. That is an awful lot. Now we cut a 1/2-inch thick slice, and eat one-fourth of the slice." They've added salads to their meals, eliminated most canned foods—Sue can taste the preservatives in them—and enjoy her homemade vegetable soup often.

- What changes can I make to adjust for unexpected events—parties, family gatherings, travel, and illness?

- How can I stay motivated? Where can I learn more? What classes can I take? What cookbooks or other books can I find?

- How can I deal with resistance to change or other roadblocks my family might put up?

The meal plan you and your dietitian come up with will probably be based on standards of nutrition endorsed by the ADA. A basic meal plan, adjusted to fit your needs, looks like this:

- Daily calorie intake should be appropriate to achieve and maintain a healthy weight.

- Fiber intake of at least 25 grams each day.

- Carbohydrate, preferably in the form of high-fiber, complex carbohydrates like whole grains, dried peas and beans, and fresh fruits and vegetables, should make up about 55 percent of your calories each day.

- Protein, preferably from sources like lean meats and cheeses and other dairy products, should make up about 15 percent of your calories each day.

- Fat, preferably from sources low in saturated fat and cholesterol, should make up no more than 30 percent of your calories each day.

- Planned snacks.

Learning the Six Food Groups

The ADA, together with The American Dietetic Association, created a system of meal planning for healthy eating that categorizes foods into six groups. Foods within a group have a similar nutritional makeup; this means that they are composed of similar proportions of protein, carbohydrate, and fat. These proportions vary greatly from group to group. The six food groups are Starch/Bread, Meat and Meat Substitutes, Vegetable, Fruit, Fat, and Milk. Learning to think of how each food you eat fits into one or more of these groups is the first step to healthier eating.

89

The key to using the meal planning system is portion size. Each serving of a food in the Starch/Bread category, for instance, has about the same number of calories and the same amount of carbohydrate, protein, and fat as do other servings of food in that group. You may substitute one serving of a particular Starch/Bread item for one serving of any other Starch/Bread item. These lists are called the *Exchange Lists for Meal Planning* because of this feature.

Meals are built around servings from the different groups. For example, lunch might be composed of 2 Starch/Bread servings, 2 Meat or Meat Substitute servings, 1 Vegetable serving, 1 Fruit serving, and 1 Fat serving. Such a lunch could look like this:

A broiled open-face sandwich made of

    2 1-inch slices Italian bread (2 Starch/Bread servings)

    2 oz. part-skim mozzarella cheese (2 Meat Substitute servings)

    Zucchini, tomato, onion, and green pepper slices (1 Vegetable serving)

    Garlic powder, basil, and black pepper (Free food)

    1 small banana (1 Fruit serving)

    1 Tbsp. reduced-calorie margarine (1 Fat serving)

Your meal plan will help you

- Replace refined and processed sugars—those used in cookies, crackers, cakes, syrups, jellies, and cereals—with those found naturally in fruits, vegetables, and milk.

- Eat more complex carbohydrates, including whole grains like oats, whole wheat, and brown rice; legumes such as peas and beans; whole-grain or vegetable pastas; whole-grain bread; corn; and low-sugar breakfast cereals.

- Add both soluble and insoluble fiber slowly.

- Reduce the amount of fat and cholesterol by choosing lean cuts of meat (such as tenderloin), skinless poultry, and fish and avoiding liver, high-fat cheeses, whole-milk products, and fried foods.

- Lower the sodium you consume by avoiding processed meats, salty snacks, and fast foods.

To learn more about healthy food choices, see Chapter 6.

Sugar and Artificial Sweeteners

Keeping the amount of refined sugars you eat low will be challenging. Hidden sugars go by many names: high-fructose corn syrup, honey, sucrose, lactose, maltose, dextrose, molasses, cane sugar, cane sweetener, invert sugar, turbinado sugar, raw sugar, brown sugar, sorghum, xylitol, and sorbitol.

WEIGHT-LOSS CLINICS—PROMISES, PROMISES

If you are considering a weight-loss clinic, proceed with caution. Consult your primary care physician before you begin.

The program should include medical supervision. An MD should be available for consultation with you. You should also be monitored by your primary care physician and the staff of the weight-loss clinic. A physician with a specialty in nutrition or bariatric medicine (the treatment of overweight people, although not specifically overweight people with diabetes) will be more sensitive to the issues you face. Ask the physician whether he or she specializes or has a special interest in diabetes.

Look for programs that also have a psychologist available to work with the staff to provide support or therapy. Look for a counselor who is licensed by the state and has at least a master's degree in psychology. Also, look for a program that has an exercise physiologist.

Choose a program that has

- Education—teaching you about proper nutrition and healthy food choices.

- Evaluation and maintenance—you should receive regular follow-up visits.

- An exercise program—increasing your physical activity, even modestly, will help you lose weight and maintain your weight loss.

- Behavior modification—helping you learn techniques for replacing old habits with new, healthier choices.

Learn to spot them. Also note that many of the low-fat or nonfat baked goods contain a lot of sugar.

The good news is that if your diet is well-rounded and low in fat, generous amounts of carbohydrate, including foods made with sugar, are in order. Once your overall diet no longer contains much of the high-fat, sugary snacks you used to eat, there's a good chance you'll stop missing them.

Artificial sweeteners may make your meal plan more livable. However, as with most foods, remember that moderation is the best approach. The available artificial sweeteners are aspartame (Equal or Nutrasweet), acesulfame-K (Sweet One or Sunette), or saccharin (Sweet 'n Low, Sugar Twin, or Sweet 10). More are being developed. For baking, use sweeteners made of acesulfame-K or saccharin, which don't break down in high heat. The ADA approves the use of these artificial sweeteners but cautions pregnant women to avoid heavy use of saccharin.

YOUR EXERCISE PLAN

Sweating, huffing, puffing, red-in-the face, uncomfortable, do-I-have-to exercise? It may be the last thing you want to think about. Adjusting to a meal plan may be tough enough. Now you're supposed to become some kind of fitness nut? Or, maybe you've always been an active sort. Now that you have diabetes, do you have to slow down?

The value of exercise cannot be overestimated. The ADA considers an exercise program part of the treatment of type II diabetes.

Your exercise of choice doesn't have to be strenuous, expensive, or inconvenient. Walking is the perfect example; you can walk anywhere, nearly any time. It's aerobic, and it takes no special skills. What is aerobic? Aerobic exercise means that you are increasing your body's consumption of oxygen appreciably. When the weather is unpleasant, try walking in a nearby shopping mall. The cost is minimal—the price of a good pair of walking shoes. The next time you're tempted to circle the parking lot looking for a space close to an entrance, go ahead and park further out. Use the time to walk instead.

Regular aerobic exercise can help lower blood pressure and reduce your risk of heart disease in addition to improving your outlook on life. Muscle toning can help increase your stamina and improve your overall appearance. Making exercise a part of your regular routine can help you cope better with the stresses and challenges of your life. It's a great way to expand your social horizons.

Before You Begin

It's important to know that exercise can pose risks to people with certain complications of diabetes. Before you start any exercise program, discuss your plans with your health-care team. You and your primary care physician may want to work with an exercise physiologist or physical therapist to tailor an exercise program to your needs.

You need your physician's go-ahead to begin an exercise program. If you are over 40, this means you need a thorough medical examination—head to feet—before you start. The exam should include tests for high blood pressure; nerve damage; and kidney, eye, and heart disease. If you are older than 35, having an electrocardiogram is the simplest and least expensive way to detect heart disease. Your feet need a good once over, too.

Safe, Effective Exercising

The most important guideline is to find an exercise routine that fits your general physical condition and your lifestyle. Doing too much too fast, or doing more than you are capable of, can lead to injuries that could keep you from doing anything at all.

Each time you exercise, take time to warm up and cool down at the beginning and end of your routine. Warm-up exercising includes low-intensity movements as you gradually work up your level of exertion. Cooling down should work in reverse. Both should contain gentle stretching movements and plenty of deep breathing.

To get the most from your time output, do aerobic exercises. Aerobic exercise benefits your heart, lungs, and muscles. It's the best way to use up calories for a weight-loss program.

Determining how hard and how frequently you should exercise safely might require the help of an exercise specialist. Some people will get the most benefit from exercising each day for 20 to 30 minutes. Others will get where they want by working out three times a week. Everyone's needs are different.

If you take oral medication or insulin, discuss the effects of your medication schedule with your health-care team to head off any unexpected blood glucose swings. Know what to do

93

when faced with very high or very low blood glucose levels before or after exercising.

You'll want to take good care of yourself when you exercise. It's important for you to

- Wear proper footwear and any other protective equipment you may need (such as safety goggles for racquetball, a bicycle helmet for cycling).

- Avoid exercising in extremely hot or cold conditions.

- Check your feet every day and after each exercise session.

- Avoid exercising when your diabetes is in poor control (blood glucose over 240 mg/dl).

Steps to Success

Just as no single meal plan works for everyone with diabetes, no exercise regimen works across the board. You'll want to individualize your program so that you'll stick with it.

- **Convenience**: make it easy on yourself. Choose a class or exercise workout that you can do with a minimum of travel time and preparation. Find something that you can fit easily into your daily routine. Good examples are walking, cycling on a stationary bike at home, or joining a neighborhood exercise class. How can you fit something into your daily routine? Some people find walking at lunch time convenient. For others, signing up for an exercise class helps them feel committed.

- **Cost**: select an activity that won't cost you a fortune in special equipment, clothes, or fees. Consider second-hand equipment or a jogging trampoline (usually around $50) in front of the television. On the other hand, making an investment in a new pair of shoes just for exercise might motivate you to use them.

- **Classes**: many communities now offer a variety of exercise classes. Ask at community centers, churches, and schools (price is usually reasonable, too). Group support can really help. These can range from in-pool aerobics to water walking to low-impact aerobics. Be cautious, however. Not all exercise classes are equally good. Go observe or try out a class before signing up; the end of a session is a good time to do this for free. Look for instructors who are certified and have cardiopulmonary resuscitation (CPR) training.

Classes should include a warm-up phase, an aerobic phase, a cool-down phase, and stretching. Instructors should have students do heart-rate monitoring (counting your pulse) during class. Good teachers modify their routines for students' differing abilities.

EXERCISING CONTROL

Harold Dixon was diagnosed with diabetes after suffering a heart attack at age 63. After the heart attack, he took off 90 pounds and began to feel better. But he became depressed about having diabetes and having to take insulin injections. He decided to try a class of water and low-impact aerobics for people with type II diabetes at his local YMCA. Like others with type II diabetes who joined the Las Vegas program, Dixon found that exercise so improved his condition that he could maintain normal blood glucose levels without medication. Now, he says, "I can 'exercise' control over diabetes while physically upgrading my whole body."

When Don Smith, now 87, first came to the water aerobics class, his blood glucose level was so high (385 mg/dl) that he was not allowed to join the group. (People with extremely high glucose levels can actually increase their blood glucose even higher by exercising. It is important to know your glucose level before exercising and to discuss any exercise program with your physician before you start. Generally, it not considered advisable to exercise with blood glucose levels over 240 mg/dl.)

Don and the exercise counselors explored some potential causes of his high glucose level, such as lack of information or poor diet and discussed ways he could control his blood glucose. He later admitted how much the information had helped him. "What I ate in the evening had much to do with my glucose level the following morning. I adjusted my diet and came in the next time boasting a 290 mg/dl reading. After the exercise, my level dropped to about 260. Over the next six weeks, my glucose gradually came down more and more and eventually averaged out at 195 on arrival, dropping to 150 after the class."

Is It Aerobic?

Aerobic exercise helps condition your heart, lungs, and muscles through effective use of oxygen. Aerobic does not mean working yourself into a lather. Exercise can be relatively low key and still be effective. Walking and in-pool aerobics classes are two good examples. If you're thinking about aerobic dancing, look for low-impact classes or just do the low-impact version that the teacher demonstrates. Low impact is kinder and gentler on your joints.

To get a conditioning effect from your aerobic exercise, you have to exert yourself enough to get your heart beating in the "target" range and sustain it for at least 20 minutes three times a week.

You should discuss your "target heart rate" for exercise with your primary care physician. A maximum capacity can be calulated for you. Then you determine whether you want to work at 60, 70, or 80 percent of that capacity. The following formula is frequently used to calculate target heart rates:

220 − your age = maximum heart rate
    × 0.60 = minimum working heart rate
    × 0.80 = maximum working heart rate

Using this formula, if you are 55 years old,

220 − 55 = 165 beats per minute
165 × 0.60 = 99 beats per minute
165 × 0.80 = 132 beats per minute

This means, your target heart rate range during exercise is between 99 and 132 beats per minute.

Be sure to discuss your target heart range with your physician. If you are very overweight, at first you may be instructed to work with lower target heart range—say 50 to 60 percent of your maximum. You'll also want to practice taking a heart rate with your doctor. Then practice at home before trying to take it while exercising. Here's one way:

- Find your pulse at your wrist or on the front of your neck just below one of your jawbones.

(Cont.)

(Cont.)

- Watching the sweep hand of a watch, count the number heart beats in six seconds, starting with zero.

- Multiply this by 10 to give you the number of beats per minute.

For example, 8 heart beats $\times$ 10 = 80 beats per minute. You can compare this to your working heart rate range to see if you are walking briskly enough or swimming steadily.

Remember: easy does it. Beginners should exercise at the lower end of their target heart rate range. Start gradually and build up slowly. For example, suppose you've been sedentary for some time. You may want to start by walking for five minutes at a time and gradually build up to 15 or 20 minutes three or four times a week. Again, consult your health-care team about the best exercise program for you.

- **Goals:** set reasonable, realistic, and measurable goals. Work with your health-care team on this. Break the goals down, so you can see your achievements. For example, if you're beginning walking for fitness, a starting goal might be getting out three times a week for one month. At the end of one month you can evaluate your progress and possibly revise your program.

- **Rewards:** give yourself a well-earned pat on the back when your reach your goal. For example, you could plan to reward yourself with a new warm-up suit or a pair of hand weights when you complete four months of walking.

- **Enjoyment:** think about what you enjoy and incorporate that into your exercise program. If you're the social type, chances are you'll enjoy the camaraderie and support of an exercise class. Do you value time alone? Swimming laps might be for you. Are you a bird watcher? Nature hikes offer exercise and beautiful surroundings.

- **Support:** try the buddy system. Find someone to exercise with; ask a friend or relative to take a class with you.

Making the commitment to meet someone for walks can help get you out the door.

- **Learning:** read up on fitness. When you've found an activity you enjoy, keep yourself inspired by reading articles, books, or personal accounts of others who enjoy your chosen sport.

- **Novelty:** try something new. Are your becoming bored with the same old exercise routine? Learn a new skill. Try something you've always been curious about. Many communities offer a range of fitness classes from fencing to lap swimming to karate. Cross-training might be for you: research has shown that the best way to achieve overall fitness is to do different exercises instead of the same ones day after day. Try basketball or racquetball one day, swimming one day, aerobic dancing for two days, and walking on the other days. Pedal your bike once in a while, too. Have you considered walking a round of golf or trying the latest version of outdoor roller skates?

YOUR EYE-CARE PLAN

You've already learned about the importance of regular eye examinations for people with diabetes. Early detection and treatment of eye problems are your best defense against a serious loss of vision.

Help protect your vision by working to keep your blood glucose levels in the normal range and keeping your blood pressure under control. Uncontrolled high blood pressure can complicate eye problems.

It's important to know that even if your vision seems fine, eye disease may be present. On the positive side, today there are effective treatments for many eye problems, including such commonly occurring conditions as cataracts, glaucoma, and diabetic retinopathy (disease of the blood vessels of the retina, the nervous tissue at the back of the eye that forms visual images).

How Often Should I Get My Eyes Checked?

The ADA recommends

- A comprehensive eye and visual examination by an eye doctor at the time of diabetes diagnosis.

■ After your initial exam, you should have yearly follow-up exams. If problems are detected, you may need more frequent exams.

■ If you have diabetes and are pregnant or planning a pregnancy, you should have an eye exam. All women with diabetes who are pregnant should have an eye exam by an ophthalmologist during the first trimester.

What Should My Eye Exam Include?

During a baseline ophthalmic examination, your eye doctor should

■ Take a history of your visual symptoms—tell him or her about any eye surgery, eye disease, or disturbances of vision you have had.

■ Measure your visual acuity (how well you see) with a chart and intraocular pressure (test for glaucoma).

■ Dilate your pupils with eye drops and perform an ophthalmoscopic examination through dilated pupils. An ophthalmoscope is the instrument that allows a doctor to look into the eye and see the retina. Your eye doctor should check for signs of diabetic retinopathy as well as for other diseases of the retina and the optic nerve not necessarily due to diabetes.

How Do I Select an Eye-Care Specialist?

If you are looking for a new eye doctor, ask your primary care physician for a referral. You'll want to choose an eye-care specialist who is knowledgeable about diabetes and the eye problems associated with the disease.

Ophthalmologists are MDs who specialize in diseases of the eye. Ophthalmologists are trained to treat eye problems both medically and surgically.

Retina specialists are ophthalmologists who have special training in diagnosis and treatment of diseases of the retina.

Optometrists are trained in examining the eye for any problems, such as how well your eyes focus, farsightedness, and nearsightedness, and in prescribing corrective lenses or eye exercises. Optometrists are not medical doctors and cannot perform surgery and, in some states, cannot prescribe medications for eye disease.

Because you have diabetes, the ADA recommends you see an ophthalmologist for diagnosis and treatment if you have

- Unexplained visual problems (spots, "floaters," or cobwebs in the field of vision; blurred or distorted vision; blind spots; eye pain or persistent redness).

- Deterioration in visual acuity (visual ability to read books or traffic signs, or to distinguish familiar objects).

- Increased intraocular pressure (a warning sign of glaucoma). Some internists, family practitioners, and optometrists test for this.

- Any abnormality of the retina. Internists, family practitioners, and optometrists should test for this but refer serious problems to ophthalmologists.

- Retinopathy, the leaking of blood vessels that supply the retina, the main cause of blindness in people with diabetes.

Can I Develop Retinopathy?

Doctors aren't sure yet precisely what factors are associated with developing retinopathy. The length of time you have had diabetes and your blood glucose levels, blood pressure, and genetic makeup all seem to play a part.

The longer you have diabetes, the more likely you are to have retinopathy. About 50 percent of non-insulin-taking people have some degree of retinopathy after 20 years with diabetes. However, only a small fraction, less than 10 percent, have proliferative retinopathy, the overproduction of new blood vessels in the retina that can most seriously diminish sight.

Your best bets for avoiding trouble?

- Have periodic eye exams by an eye-care specialist familiar with retinopathy and eye problem associated with diabetes.

- Call your primary care physician if you notice changes in your vision, but don't panic. Highs and lows in your blood glucose level may cause temporary blurring in your vision.

- Keep your blood glucose levels under control.

- Get your blood pressure checked regularly and work to keep it in the healthy range.

Your Dental Care Plan

It may seem odd that taking care of your teeth and mouth is an important healthy habit if you have diabetes, but the fact is that dental care is especially important.

Most Americans over the age of 40 have some form of gum (periodontal) disease, ranging from mild gum inflammation (gingivitis) to severe periodontal infection. People with diabetes are at high risk for developing periodontitis, the more severe form of gum disease. Periodontal disease is often more frequent and more severe in people with diabetes and tends to appear at an earlier age.

This may have to do with the changes in blood vessels that diabetes causes. In your mouth, as well as elsewhere in your body, blood vessels perform the work of carrying both oxygen and nutrients to the cells and removing waste products. Some evidence shows that diabetes causes blood vessels to thicken, slowing down this flow of oxygen, vital nutrients, and waste removal. In the mouth this can weaken the resistance of your gum and bone tissues to infection.

In addition, many kinds of bacteria thrive on sugars, like glucose. If your diabetes is poorly controlled, high glucose levels in your mouth fluids may encourage the growth of harmful germs and set the stage for gum infection.

The good news is if you keep your diabetes well controlled, you face no more risk of gingivitis or periodontitis than the population in general. However, if your diabetes is poorly controlled, your chances of infection increase.

Caring for Your Teeth

Your first line of defense against gum disease is brushing and flossing thoroughly every day and working to achieve normal-range blood glucose levels. Some tips on brushing and flossing follow below. Ask your dentist or dental hygienist for more specifics on your personal tooth-care routine.

- Keep your blood glucose levels under control. This is the next most important step you can take to prevent tooth and gum problems. A severe gum infection can raise blood glucose levels and make controlling your diabetes harder. Once an infection starts, diabetes can delay healing, and long-term infections can lead to tooth loss.

■ See your dentist at least every six months. Tell your dentist that you have diabetes. Your dentist or dental hygienist will clean your teeth. Then, your dentist will check for any spots that require special attention, diagnose bleeding gums, look for any detachment of gum tissue from the teeth. Ask your dentist or hygienist to show you proper flossing and brushing techniques.

■ Brushing helps remove plaque (a sticky film containing millions of bacteria) from your teeth. Brush at least twice a day, carefully and not too vigorously. Use a soft nylon brush with rounded ends on its bristles. Proper brushing technique includes these steps: brushing at a 45-degree angle where the teeth meet the gums; next, brushing the outside surfaces of all teeth with short back-and-forth strokes; following the same approach for the backs of teeth and chewing surfaces; and it's even a good idea to brush the rough upper surface of the tongue.

■ Use dental floss once a day to remove bacteria from between the teeth. Your dentist or dental hygienist can show you how to get to some of the harder to reach spots. Special floss holders and various types of floss are available to make flossing easier. Ask your dentist or hygienist to check your brushing and flossing technique.

■ Check with your dentist if you notice that your gums bleed while you are eating or brushing your teeth. You may be able to catch an infection in the beginning stages.

When to See Your Dentist

Besides your regular checkups, any of these symptoms of gum disease are signals to see your dentist:

■ Gums bleed when you brush your teeth.

■ Red, swollen, or tender gums.

■ Gums have pulled away from your teeth.

■ Pus appears between your teeth and gums when the gums are pressed.

■ Teeth are becoming loose or changing position.

■ Any change in the way your partial dentures fit.

- Any change in the way your teeth fit together when you bite.

- Persistent bad breath or a bad taste in your mouth.

Before You Have Surgery

Check with your primary care physician before treatment for periodontal disease. Your dentist or periodontist (gum specialist) should consult with your physician before gum surgery to learn about your general condition. Your physician will probably put you on an antibiotic before surgery to prevent infection.

If your diabetes is poorly controlled, you'll want to delay treatment for periodontal disease until you can bring your blood glucose levels into better control. This should not take too long to accomplish. However, an acute infection, such as an abscess, should be treated immediately.

103

SWEET SLIP-UP

It took a while for Larry Miller to be concerned about having diabetes. Eventually his doctor convinced him to start taking care of himself better after a time when his blood glucose level rose too high.

Larry, a writer for television, was working on a pilot for a stunt show called *Fun House*. Some of the stunts used licorice, marshmallows, and other sugary treats. Larry indulged more than he should have. Later he went to his doctor and had his blood glucose tested. Larry's doctor got tough with him and reemphasized that his eating habits were increasing the risk for complications. "I'm glad my doctor scared me before anything did happen," says Larry, who hasn't suffered any serious problems because of his diabetes.

Since the *Fun House* binge, Larry has lost 30 pounds and wants to lose more. His goal is to have his doctor take him off the oral medication that Larry uses to control his diabetes. Chances are good that if Larry can lose the weight and keep it off, he'll also be able to stay off the medication, emergencies aside.

If you have periodontal surgery, diabetes may slow your healing. With good medical and dental care, your chances of complications are no greater than those of someone without diabetes. Once the periodontal infection is treated, you may even find your blood glucose level is easier to control.

If dental work has left your mouth tender, eating may pose a challenge. Consider filling your meal plan with some of the liquid or soft foods listed below in "Your Sick Day Plan." A special call to your dietitian may be in order.

YOUR SKIN-CARE PLAN

You've already learned that having diabetes means that you are at greater risk for infections. Unfortunately, the skin you're in offers a tempting target. Diabetes may cause some special skin problems. There are two things you can do to help prevent these from occurring:

- Keep your diabetes well controlled.

- Practice good skin care.

Feet First

Because you have diabetes, you need to check the skin on your feet daily. Poor blood circulation in the feet and legs is common in people with type II diabetes. This makes the skin thin and easily broken. If you have nerve disease (neuropathy), you may not feel a cut or blister on your foot. A small cut or blister could become infected, and you may not feel any warning pain. Also, feet may become dry, and the skin may crack. If your feet are an area of concern to you, you may want to ask your primary care physician to recommend a podiatrist. See below for more on how to care for your feet.

The Rest of Your Skin

If your diabetes is not well controlled, you may find yourself more susceptible to skin infections. Small cuts or breaks in the skin allow bacteria to enter and infection to start. Bacterial infections can cause redness, pain, and swelling.

Fungus can also cause skin infections. These are usually itchy rashes in the moist areas of skin folds, such as the armpits or between the toes. But they can also occur just about anywhere, most of the time as raised, peeling patches. Common fungal infections are jock itch, athlete's feet, ringworm (a ring-shaped itchy patch on the skin), and vaginal itching.

Some people with diabetes get special skin conditions called diabetic dermopathy. Symptoms include sores that do not go away or a reddish-yellowish rash, usually on the lower legs and shins. If you notice these symptoms, see your primary care physician. You can get treatment.

In rare instances, people who have an allergic reaction to oral diabetes medications or insulin injections may develop skin problems. If you develop a rash or notice bumps or pits in the skin near an injection site, see your primary care physician.

Caring for Your Skin

By taking good care of your skin, you can stop skin problems before they start.

- Keep your skin clean and dry. Pay attention to the skin folds (armpits, groin, and under the breasts) where fungal infections can occur.

- Avoid very hot baths and showers. If your skin is dry, skip the bubble bath. Use a superfatted soap such as Dove, Basis, Keri, or Oilatum. Afterward, you may need to use an oil-in-water skin cream such as Lubriderm or Alpha-Keri.

- Prevent dry skin. Scratching dry, itchy skin can lead to breaks in the skin. These can turn into bacterial infections. Try using only mild soaps or soaps with creams or oils; use oils, lotions, and creams regularly—especially after bathing; moisturize your skin to prevent chapping—especially in cold or windy weather. Don't put moisturizing creams or lotions **between** your toes because this creates excessive moisture and may lead to infection.

- Use mild shampoos, and avoid feminine hygiene sprays and scented soaps. If you have questions about the use of feminine hygiene products, ask your primary care physician. Consider wearing only all-cotton underwear, which gives improved air circulation over other types of underwear. All of this advice is good even if you don't have diabetes.

- Treat cuts quickly. For minor cuts, clean the area with soap and water; then, lightly dress with a cotton gauze square secured with a gauze knot or tape placed on the gauze only (not touching the skin). **Do not** use antiseptics such as Mercurochrome, alcohol, or iodine because they may irritate the skin. Ask your physician before you use antibiotic creams or ointments. For any signs or symptoms of infection (such as redness, swelling, pus, or pain), severe cuts, or burns, get medical help immediately.

■ Ask for help if you need it. If you are prone to skin problems, ask your doctor about adding a dermatologist (an MD trained in diseases of the skin) to your health-care team.

YOUR FOOT-CARE PLAN

Ordinary foot problems can quickly escalate into serious trouble and lead to painful complications when you have type II diabetes. This is especially true if you have poor circulation or nerve damage in your lower extremities. You can help protect your feet by following a regular foot-care routine.

As a part of any visit, your primary care physician should check your feet carefully. Routinely remove your shoes and socks to remind both of you to look. During each complete physical exam, your doctor will check for pulses, reflexes, sensation, calluses, infections, and sores. These should be checked anytime you have a foot complaint.

Common Foot Problems

Bring any concerns you have about your feet to the attention of your primary care physician. You may need to be referred to a podiatrist.

■ **Dry, scaly skin.** Diabetes can cause changes in the skin of your foot. At times your foot may become very dry; the skin may peel and crack. If the skin on your foot becomes dry, try the following treatment. After bathing, dry your feet. Take care to dry between the toes. Seal in the moisture that remains by applying an extremely thin coating of lubricant. Good choices are plain petroleum jelly, unscented hand creams, or aqueous lanolin. Do this twice a day. A word of caution: do not put the lubricant, oils, or creams **between** your toes. This creates excessive moisture and can lead to infection.

■ **Calluses**. Daily gentle use of pumice stones can help keep calluses under control. However, never try to cut calluses or corns yourself. Home surgery almost always makes problems worse, especially if you have impaired vision or dexterity. Let your physician or podiatrist handle the cutting. Do not use chemical agents to remove calluses or corns. These are too harsh for your feet. Cracks developing in calluses can be dangerous because they allow bacteria to penetrate and cause infection. Treating this is best handled by your podiatrist.

Our feet evolved to carry most of the weight on the bones of the big toe. When weight bearing is faulty, calluses form. If you have a callus, consider asking your podiatrist or physician about shoe inserts to distribute your weight onto your feet properly.

■ **Foot ulcers**. Ulcers on the feet are open wounds that are deep and can have dying tissue beneath the surface of the wound. The most likely places for a foot ulcer to develop are over the ball of the foot and on the bottom of the big toe. Poorly fitting shoes can also lead to ulcers on the sides of the feet. Even though you may not feel any pain from an ulcer, you need to get immediate medical attention. Walking on an ulcer can cause it to become larger and the infection to penetrate deeper into the tissues. You can help avoid this problem by wearing properly fitting shoes and socks, wearing new shoes a few hours at a time, and checking for pebbles or other objects before you put your shoes on. Do not use worn-out footwear. Do not wear socks more than once without washing them.

■ **Neuropathy**. Diabetic neuropathy can lead to a loss of sensation in your feet. (Interestingly, neuropathy can also result in foot pain.) This means that a foot injury can go unnoticed. If you develop neuropathy, your best line of foot defense is regular inspections. Check your feet daily for any changes. Check the insides of your shoes for rough edges and foreign objects. Never walk barefoot, even in tempting situations like at the beach, around the swimming pool, or at home.

■ **Poor circulation**. If you have poor circulation, your feet may feel cold. The best way to treat your cold feet is to wear warm socks, even to bed. Do not use hot water bottles or heating pads and never soak your feet in hot water—if you've lost some sensation in your feet, you could easily be burned. Avoid activities that will restrict the blood flow to your feet like smoking or sitting with your legs crossed. Do not wear garters, which can put pressure on blood vessels. Exercise is good for poor circulation. Just walking helps to stimulate the blood flow to your feet. Of course, you need to check with your physician before adding any form of exercise to your diabetes care plan.

Caring for Your Feet

Check your feet and toes daily, take all foot injuries seriously, and, when necessary, get prompt medical attention. Chances are good you'll be able to steer clear of serious problems that could lead to amputation of part of your foot.

- Inspect your feet and between your toes daily. You can use a mirror to help see the bottom of your feet. If your vision is impaired, have a family member examine your feet daily.

- Trim your toenails straight across.

- Wear properly fitting shoes. Do not expect to have to "break in" new shoes. Although almost all new shoes are stiff at the start and mold to your feet with wear, this is different from buying the wrong size and trying to break them in. A podiatrist can help you with shoe selection.

YOUR SICK DAY PLAN

Getting sick can ruin your carefully assembled self-care routine. Unexpected vomiting or nausea can play havoc with your meal plan and lead to dangerous dehydration, and your body's natural defenses to illness can send your blood glucose levels upward.

When you're sick your body is stressed. To deal with this stress, your body releases hormones that normally help the body fight disease. Unfortunately, these also elevate blood glucose levels and counteract the glucose-lowering effects of insulin. Sickness can cause your diabetes to go out of control. Extremely high blood glucose levels can lead to a serious condition called hyperglycemic hyperosmolar coma, especially in elderly people

---

LAUGHING AT IT

Diabetes demands major lifestyle changes. Food and diet become projects. Food is portioned out in terms of exchanges. A Meat exchange is about 1 ounce. Have you ever seen 1 ounce of anything? Postage stamps are bigger. I used to wipe out a few 1 ouncers before even eating dinner.

There is a category of exchanges called "Free Food." You can eat all the herbs you desire. Fresh parsley could become the new pig-out food. Cabbage is another. I've taken stock in the Nappa Cabbage Company. After all, 14 million possible customers raise a lot of potenial.

Exercise is a new experience—and I'll admit going to the gym is a little discouraging. Entering the "Y," I noticed one young lady on a stationary bicycle. I decided to try some leg presses. The machine was being used by a woman doing a number of sets. When she finished, I subtly moved the pin from the 250-pound weight to the 10-pound weight and pretended to exercise with the same vigor.

Next was the stationary bike. Peggy Pump was still pedaling away. She even had her feet taped to the pedals for maximum effort. The indicator said 8. I climbed onto the second bike and eventually got through 20 minutes. For a brief moment of glory, the needle on my bike registered a 2.

Staggering off the bike, I went to the locker room, had a long shower, dressed, and left for home. Peggy was still pedaling away. She's probably still there.

—*Dan MacLachlan, Akron, Ohio*

---

with type II diabetes. You can see why you need to discuss sick day strategies with your health-care team before illness strikes. You, your primary care physician, and your diabetes educator and/or dietitian together can work out strategies that will help you handle common illnesses such as colds and flu.

You need to have the answers to these questions for your sick day plan:

- When to call the doctor.

- How to handle blood glucose testing.

- Whether you should perform urine ketone testing. Ketones are produced when fat instead of glucose is used as a source of energy, which can happen when illness sends glucose levels soaring. Their presence in urine indicates that the body is not getting the insulin it needs (they also appear if your doctor places you on a very-low-calorie diet). Most people with type II diabetes do not need to monitor urine ketone levels.

- Medication changes that might be necessary. Remember, only your primary care physician can tell you when and how to change your insulin or oral medication dosage.

- Whether to have antinausea suppositories or pills on hand and when to take them.

- Foods and fluids to take during your illness.

When to Call Your Doctor

The answer to this question will depend on your illness, your diabetes control, and the general state of your health. Discuss this with your primary care physician. General guidelines might include calling when

- An illness has continued for one or two days without improvement.

- Vomiting or diarrhea has continued for longer than six hours.

- Self-testing shows moderate to large amounts of ketones in your urine.

- You are taking insulin, and your blood glucose levels continue to be over 240 mg/dl after taking two or three supplemental doses of Regular insulin as prearranged with your doctor.

- You are taking insulin, and hypoglycemia is occurring (blood glucose is under 60 mg/dl).

- You are taking oral diabetes medication and your premeal blood glucose levels are 240 mg/dl or more for more than 24 hours.

- You have signs of extreme hyperglycemia, dehydration, or loss of mental competence.

When you do call, your physician will depend on you to have some information ready. Keep records during your illness so that you and your doctor can evaluate how sick you are **and** keep track of your progress getting well.

Here are some things your doctor will want to know:

- Your blood glucose level and your urine ketone results.

- How much and what type of insulin or diabetes pills you have taken and when you have taken them.

- Other medications you have taken.

- How long you've been sick.

- Your temperature (make sure you have a fever thermometer).

- How well you can take foods and fluids.

- If you have lost weight while sick. (This can be a sign of dehydration.)

- Any other symptoms you may have.

If you are treated by someone other than your regular physician, be sure to tell him or her about your diabetes.

Keep the phone numbers of your primary care physician, diabetes educator, dietitian, health-care clinic, and hospital emergency room handy. Know where to reach members of your health-care team or their back ups on weekends, holidays, and evenings.

Self-Monitoring

In general, during an illness you may need to monitor your blood glucose level every three to four hours. Some people, including pregnant women, may need to monitor more often. Ask your doctor how much you should monitor and when. You will also need to check for ketones if your blood glucose level is more than 240 mg/dl.

Medications

You'll need to discuss this promptly with your health-care team. Only your physician can tell you when to change your medications. When you are sick,

- Do not stop taking your insulin or oral diabetes medications. Even if you can't keep food down, your body needs insulin to counter the high levels of glucose that illness produces.

- If you take insulin, make sure you understand your physician's previous instructions about any additional quantities or different types of insulin and any changes in times of injections. When in doubt, call sooner rather than later.

- If you take oral diabetes medications, take your medication if you can. Sometimes on sick days you may temporarily need to take insulin. Follow your doctor's instructions.

When you are sick, you may take some additional medications. Check the label of any nonprescription medication for sugar content. Although many cough medications and throat lozenges contain sugar, taking one or two lozenges or a teaspoon or even a tablespoon of liquid medication is usually not dangerous. However, you may prefer to look for sugar-free preparations (ask your pharmacist). You may want to keep a small supply of sick day medications on hand that have been approved for your use by your primary care physician.

SHOULD I GET A FLU SHOT?

Doctors generally advise all people who have diabetes to get a flu shot. However, there are pros and cons to having the vaccine, so discuss this with your primary care physician. You can also ask about the Pneumococcus vaccine to prevent bacterial pneumonia.

Foods and Fluids

It is important to watch out for dehydration during sickness. Discuss specifics with your doctor and/or dietitian. In general, you should

- Prepare a sick day meal plan before you ever become ill. You may want to set aside a small area of your cupboard for those foods and liquids you use during illness such as diet and regular soft drinks, chicken soup, bouillon cubes, broth, applesauce, and gelatin.

- Try to follow your normal meal plan. You can supplement it with caffeine-free fluids, such as broth, diet and regular

SOFT AND LIQUID FOODS FOR SICK DAY MEAL PLANS	
1 serving of Starch/Bread:	1/2 cup mashed potatoes
	1/3 cup cooked rice
	6 saltine crackers
	1/3 cup no-sugar frozen yogurt
	1/4 cup sherbet
	1 cup soup with rice or noodles
1 serving of Fruit:	1/2 cup applesauce
	1/2 cup low-sugar canned fruit
	1 frozen fruit juice bar
	1/2 cup fruit juice
1 serving of Milk:	1 cup creamed soup
	1/2 cup baked custard
	1/2 cup sugar-free pudding
	1 cup low-fat milk
1 serving of Meat:	1/4 cup cottage cheese
	1 ounce cheese
	1 scrambled egg
	4 ounces tofu

soft drinks, and water. Drinking fluids is important because you may be losing them, especially if you are vomiting or have a fever or diarrhea. (Regular soft drinks or other fluids with sugar or carbohydrate in them may actually help you prevent hypoglycemia if you have taken your usual dose of medication or extra insulin because of ketones in the urine and you are too nauseated to eat. Drinking 3 to 6 ounces an hour may help stabilize blood glucose levels during the most intense 6 to 12 hours of nausea.)

- Substitute sick day foods for your usual foods if nausea or vomiting make eating difficult. You'll want to talk to your dietitian about the best sick day food choices for you. You still need to stick with your basic eating plan. For instance, dinner should still include 2 servings of Starch/Bread, 2 to 3 servings of Meat or Milk, 1 or 2 servings of Vegetable, and 1 serving of Fruit exchanges. Try some of the milk options if you cannot tolerate meat. You may want to work some soft or liquid foods into your meal plan.

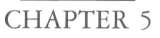

CHAPTER 5

Diabetes
Complications

A diagnosis of type II diabetes should always be accompanied by a warning about diabetes complications. These are diseases that can accompany diabetes. Some can develop quickly and dramatically, others appear after many years of diabetes. But they all have one thing in common: they are associated with and may be caused by unnaturally high blood glucose levels, or hyperglycemia.

Are you one of the thousands of people who went to the doctor for treatment of a pain or a change in your vision and came away with a diagnosis of diabetes? The nature of type II diabetes is that it sometimes shows up first as a problem caused by a diabetes complication. It is possible to have an elevated blood glucose level without being aware of it. This is why regular medical checkups are important for everyone.

When blood glucose levels remain high after eating or release of stored glucose, the excess glucose can affect many parts of the body. One of the things that happens is that your body tries to get rid of it by adding it to your urine. The kidneys work harder and more than usual. The extra glucose can attach to and coat cells and proteins; glucose-coated substances cannot do their normal jobs properly. These "sticky" cells and proteins can clog the vessels that carry blood throughout the body, disrupting the circulation. They can also affect nerve cells such that electrical messages are delayed, changed, or never reach their destination.

How your body handles long periods of hyperglycemia will be determined by your genetic makeup and the general state of your health. It's hard to predict what complications you might develop, so it's best to work to prevent them all by managing your blood glucose level, eating within your meal plan, and getting regular exercise. Diabetes complications can be treated. Some complications, such as painful nerve damage, can even disappear if several months of normal blood glucose levels are achieved.

NEUROPATHY

Nerve damage caused by high levels of blood glucose is all too common in type II diabetes. People with type II diabetes can have pain in their extremities, such as hands and feet, thighs, or face; trouble with digestion or bladder or bowel control; and impotence or other sexual dysfunction. Loss of feeling and muscular weakness are also common complaints. These can all be symptoms of diabetic neuropathy, but they may also be caused by other conditions. Losing even a portion of your ability to move in or sense the world can be disabling and disheartening.

Diabetic neuropathy basically comes in three forms: peripheral neuropathy, autonomic neuropathy, and cranial neuropathy. They are distinguished by what parts of the body are affected. Although more has yet to be discovered, the mechanisms that cause neuropathy in one part of the body are probably similar to those in other parts of the body. Somehow, hyperglycemia disrupts the ways the nerve cells normally work. This could be related to how glucose is disposed of by the cells. It is also possible that neuropathy is caused by problems in the blood supply to the nerves. Sometimes single nerves are damaged by being squeezed by surrounding tissues. Onset of neuropathy can also be related to injury.

The most common nerve disorder is peripheral neuropathy. It affects parts of the body, such as the legs and arms and sometimes the chest or abdomen, that are away from the central nervous system (the brain and spinal cord). Peripheral neuropathy can show itself in a variety of signs: shooting or stabbing pains, numbness or loss of sensation, tingling or prickling, and weakness. Sometimes, contact with things that normally do not cause pain, like bed sheets or clothes, can be painful. A loss of feeling in the feet is especially dangerous; check your footwear daily for foreign objects that may cause foot damage without you knowing it, and never go barefoot. Peripheral neuropathy affects both the sensory nerves, which collect information about your environment, and motor nerves, which allow you to consciously move your muscles. Signs of neuropathy can occur on both sides or only one side of the body.

Carpal tunnel syndrome is an example of a compression peripheral neuropathy. It occurs more often in women than men. The median nerve, which supplies the hand, can become squeezed in its passageway or "tunnel" by the carpal bones in the hand and wrist. Sensations include tingling and burning, numbness, swelling, or weakness that results in dropping things. This type of neuropathy is usually not permanent.

> ### Losing It
>
> I lost a toe because of gangrene. Was my toe green? No. When I tell people what happened, they immediately ask if my balance is all right. Why assume it was the big toe? To answer on their level, I say, "It was the little piggy that stayed home."
>
> What about the comments people make? "My brother had his toe cut off and finally his whole leg." Thank you, that's just what I need to hear.
>
> —*Dan MacLachlan, Akron, Ohio*

Less common but equally serious is autonomic neuropathy. This is damage to nerves that control unconscious function. Nerves in the autonomic system are more closely involved with your central nervous system than nerves that supply the periphery. Autonomic neuropathy can affect the digestive system by slowing the emptying of stomach contents, leading to incomplete digestion of food, and alternating between times of nausea, diarrhea, and constipation. Proper filling and emptying of the bladder can be affected. This may result in frequent urinary tract infections or incontinence. There may be a slow loss in men of the ability to achieve and maintain an erection, although desire is unchanged. Some women notice less satisfying or difficult sexual responses. The nerves supplying the heart can be affected by neuropathy. The heart may fail to change its beating pattern properly to accommodate increases in physical activity or breathing rate. Autonomic neuropathy can also affect blood pressure control. This can result in a fall in blood pressure on standing, which can lead to lightheadedness or dizziness. Autonomic neuropathy may change the way the skin functions, which can be characterized by excessive or decreased sweating and extremely dry skin.

Charcot's joint is a good example of the complex nature of diabetes complications. It is found in people who have had diabetes for many years and who are generally older than 40. It can occur in any joint, but in people with diabetes, the feet and ankles are often affected. Usually, it starts with loss of feeling in the feet. This leads to an injury, such as turning an ankle. Because of decreased sensation, the injury isn't allowed to heal properly, and muscle shrinking (atrophy) occurs.

Because autonomic neuropathy is also responsible for blood pooling in the foot, bone degeneration can occur, making the foot swollen and hot. Often, the condition becomes very server before treatment is sought. If the bones continue to break down, loss of the foot arch and deformity could make walking impossible.

Cranial neuropathy refers to problems with the nerves that supply the head and face. This type of neuropathy can cause facial pain and sometimes temporary paralysis of eye muscles or portions of the face. These symptoms usually go away without other treatment.

Treatment

Many conditions besides diabetes can promote neuropathy, so your primary care physician will be cautious in diagnosing diabetic neuropathy. For instance, drinking alcohol aggravates peripheral neuropathy. Because of the complexity of the nervous system, treatment for neuropathy needs to be directly linked to the problem. Deciding exactly what the problem is can take some time and testing. Electrical stimulation of nerves or muscles may be necessary to sort out the difficulty.

If the pain of peripheral neuropathy is severe, your physician can treat it in several ways: helping you achieve good control of your blood glucose levels, advising appropriate exercises, and prescribing topical creams or different types of oral medications. The symptoms of peripheral neuropathy can take several months to a year to disappear, and sometimes antidepressants are prescribed to help the patient deal with the anxiety and pain of this complication. Never attempt to treat neuropathy without the knowledge of your primary care physician.

Treatment for carpal tunnel syndrome includes achieving good blood glucose control, medications, or surgery to remove tissues squeezing the nerve. Getting early treatment for Charcot's joint is important and involves keeping weight off the foot and special footwear.

Several kinds of autonomic neuropathy can be effectively treated.

- Impotence due to neuropathy, sometimes also involving the circulatory system, can be treated with injections of drugs; external erection aids, such as a vacuum that pulls blood into the penis; or penis implants. The cause of impotence may be difficult to pin down. Your physician will investigate your blood glucose control, use of medications and alcohol, hormone levels, and your general mental health and happiness.

- Urinary incontinence (passing urine involuntarily) is common in women older than 50, with or without diabetes. Urine leakage can be due to childbirth, neuropathy, or infection. It usually does not indicate kidney damage. In women with diabetes, it can indicate that the nerves supplying the bladder have been damaged, which can result in failing to know when the bladder is full, the need to strain when urinating, or very slow, dribbling urination. Training in bladder control and timed urinations plus education are the first steps to treatment and can be very successful. Other treatments include learning to use a catheter, oral medications, and surgery. Fecal incontinence (passing stool involuntarily) is treated in a similar fashion: medication is given for diarrhea, along with biofeedback training.

- Sexual problems such as decreased vaginal lubrication, decreased satisfaction or desire, and painful intercourse occur in women with type II diabetes, especially in postmenopausal women. Communicating these symptoms to your primary care physician is the first step in getting help. Hormone therapy, lubricants, specific exercises, position improvement during intercourse, and referral to a mental health counselor can all be effective at increasing sexual satisfaction.

- Gastrointestinal complaints due to neuropathy are treated according to each symptom. You may have to change your eating habits, such as improving your chewing to break food into smaller particles, eating smaller meals more often, and avoiding or eating more of particular foods. Medications may be used to increase stomach secretions and contractions or reduce diarrhea. Gastrointestinal complaints are often very difficult problems that take much patience and trial and error to treat.

- Extreme low blood pressure due to changes in body position can be treated by stopping medications such as

LESSONS LEARNED LATE

Jerry Washington, better known as Wash or on the air as "the 'Bama," is a popular deejay in Washington, DC. Wash has had type II diabetes for 30 years, and he's learned first-hand how important it is to keep diabetes in control.

Unfortunately, it was a lesson he learned late in life. Wash is the first person to tell you he didn't take diabetes seriously. Complications from diabetes have contributed to the loss of his right eye and right leg.

To his credit, Wash has been very open about his diabetes. He talks about it on the air and in articles that have been written about him. "I wish I had been conscientious about my health...I ate all the wrong things and didn't take my medicine. It got to the point where sores and blisters would come on my foot and I had poor circulation. In 1985, the doctor at Walter Reed Hospital amputated my right leg."

Wash, who gets around mainly with the help of crutches, says he now takes much better control of his diabetes. "The doctor told me that if I stop drinking, he'll stop cutting. I'm in pretty good control now, not perfect control, but I'm healthier than I've been in 30 years."

diuretics, alcohol, or other drugs that may be contributing and by improving general health. In some cases, salt intake needs to be increased or sleeping position altered. There are also medications that improve low blood pressure. Rising slowly from the lying to the standing position and avoiding standing still for long periods are always useful in preventing fainting.

NEPHROPATHY

Diabetic nephropathy, damage to the kidneys because of diabetes, does not occur in all people who have diabetes. In fact, the odds are that you will not develop diabetic nephropathy. Severe damage to the kidneys due to diabetes may be less common in type II diabetes than in type I diabetes. On the other hand, kidney disease can at worst be life threatening and at the very least is a serious problem. Kidney disease can occur in the type II diabetes age-group because of other conditions, such as hypertension. Many people with type II diabetes already have hypertension at diagnosis of diabetes. Years of high blood pressure can damage the delicate filters in the kidneys, leading to less efficient waste removal from the blood.

When your type II diabetes was diagnosed, chances are good that your physician checked your urine for signs of kidney damage. Capillaries in healthy kidneys filter most everything from the blood into collecting tubules inside the kidneys. Substances needed by the body are reabsorbed in appropriate amounts from the tubules. Higher than normal levels of protein in the urine are evidence that the ability of the kidneys to filter waste products may some day become impaired.

It is not unusual for people with newly diagnosed type II diabetes to have excess protein in their urine. Unchecked hypertension and a period of hyperglycemia before diabetes was detected are two reasons for this. An interesting finding is that, for some unknown reason, higher than normal urine protein levels can predict future cardiovascular problems.

When the capillaries in the kidneys are damaged, the filters becomes less efficient at removing substances such as urea and toxic waste products. When fewer filters are functioning, the rest have to work even harder, and the damage progresses. The result is that toxins and toxic by-products remain in the blood.

Treatment

Kidney damage may be reduced or stopped from progressing by good blood glucose control and by treatment of hypertension. A diet low in protein may also be beneficial by removing the strain of filtering protein by-products. When kidney damage is already more advanced, medications to lower blood pressure will be prescribed, because normal blood pressure is essential to halting kidney damage. These drugs are all prescribed on an individual basis, due to side effects and other conditions such as coronary artery disease.

Later stages of kidney disease, when filtration is greatly impaired and the kidneys are failing, require aggressive treatment. Kidney failure is known as end-stage renal disease. Once failure occurs, there are no medications available to make the kidneys improve. Two types of therapy for kidney failure are dialysis and transplantation. Both are types of kidney replacement. Transplantation—if feasible and available—is generally more effective but requires taking drugs that prevent immune system rejection of the new kidney.

Dialysis is a method of cleaning the blood with an artificial kidney. Hemodialysis involves removing blood, passing it through a filter, and then returning the blood to the person. It is necessary to surgically prepare a site, usually an arm, to remove the unfiltered blood from an artery and return the filtered blood to a vein. The amount of blood outside the body at any time is usually small. This kind of dialysis occurs at a treatment center, unless a caregiver is extensively trained in home hemodialysis. A common side effect of this treatment is anemia (low red blood cell count), which can be effectively treated with medications or blood transfusion.

123

The other type of dialysis is called peritoneal dialysis. Instead of blood being cleansed by a machine, the abdominal cavity is used as the filtering site. A solution containing a dialysate is drained into an opening in the abdomen and allowed to collect waste products. The exchange of wastes from the blood takes place in the peritoneum, the sac-like lining of the abdominal cavity. After a few hours, the dialysate and wastes are drained out of the abdomen. This can be performed manually, by letting gravity both carry the dialysate into the cavity and drain it out again, or a machine can perform the exchange, usually overnight. The drawback to peritoneal dialysis is the risk of infection.

Kidney transplantation from a living or cadaver donor offers the best opportunity for an uninterrupted lifestyle, and results are superior to dialysis, but there are definite risks and drawbacks. A genetically near-identical donor is desirable but not essential. Good cardiovascular health is also very important. Transplantation is major surgery and is very costly. Kidney recipients must take immune system-suppressing drugs, which often have severe side effects, to prevent rejection of the new kidney.

RETINOPATHY

Diabetic retinopathy is a disease that affects the blood vessels in the retina. Like nephropathy, this disease reflects damage to very small blood vessels. Also like nephropathy, it is more common in people with type I diabetes. But many years of type II diabetes can lead to this kind of blood vessel damage just as well. Retinopathy begins when the retina receives less oxygen than needed, and blood vessels enlarge in an attempt to gain more oxygen.

Retinopathy is divided into two major types, nonproliferative and proliferative. Nonproliferative (or background) retinopathy is seen in about 20 percent of people at diagnosis of type II diabetes. This is the usually mild form of retinopathy that may result in blurred vision but almost never causes blindness. The overdilated blood vessel walls can weaken and leak blood (hemorrhage). In addition, cells that line the retinal blood vessels can be altered so that they close off the vessel. It is uncommon for people with type II diabetes to develop proliferative retinopathy, the more serious form of the disease.

In proliferative retinopathy, new blood vessels are formed in the retina. Although this may sound good, the new vessels grow without regard for what is needed, and they are fragile and rupture easily. These blood vessels can hemorrhage, leaking blood into the fluid-filled portion of the eye in front of the retina. This prevents light from reaching the retina, which disrupts vision. Blood vessel rupture can also lead to the formation of scar tissue. As scar tissue shrinks, it can pull on the retina, causing it to detach. When any part of the retina is not tight against the back of the eye, vision can be impaired (it is similar to watching a movie projected onto a white bed sheet that is moving in the breeze).

Hemorrhages may be caused by high blood pressure or increased blood pressure during exercise but may also occur while sleeping. Macular edema (swelling of the macula, the critical central portion of the retina, that gives us sharp vision for fine detail) may occur at any stage of retinopathy. It can also lead to retinal detachment. Proliferative retinopathy may also be accompanied by glaucoma, increased pressure within the eye, which can be effectively treated if detected early.

Treatment

In recent years, great advances have been made in treating diabetic retinopathy. The best known treatment for retinopathy is photocoagulation, or laser therapy. This process can help reduce the risk of visual loss and is generally effective in preventing blindness in patients who have either high-risk proliferative retinopathy (especially if accompanied by hemorrhage of new blood vessels in the retina) or severe macular edema, or both. A laser is used to make tiny burns in the retina. This destroys the abnormal blood vessels, patches up leaky vessels, and discourages formation of new fragile vessels.

When there is very extensive bleeding or the retina becomes detached, vitrectomy surgery may be needed. Vitrectomy is a

---

NOW I SEE

Naively, I once had thought myself beyond the reaches of diabetes. Denying the possibility of future problems with all the rebellious fervor I could muster, I acted as if I somehow had the power to ward off complications.

Inside this rebellion was the fear that I would not have the ability or strength to deal with complications, should they arise. I fell prey to the common misconception that blindness or neuropathy is somehow reserved for a few brave, strong individuals.

I knew that I could never face vision loss of any kind. I could never learn to live with diabetic complications or find the strength to carry on despite physical barriers. And, because of those feelings, I decided complications simply couldn't happen to me.

Then, the day came. Retinopathy was diagnosed and an emotional flood unleashed. The fabric of denial sewn together throughout 15 years of diabetic life was torn into shreds. Something that was reserved for those brave, strong few had become part of my reality.

When retinopathy started affecting my eyesight, I began to grow more introspective. The vision of myself as one of those "handicapped" people confronted me.

I realized that I am no stronger and braver than I was before. I have not been changed in any grand, significant way because of retinopathy. I don't have genetically endowed strength that rises to the surface on diagnosis of diabetic complications. I have simply been forced into a position of no return—one of creative living. After years of being too afraid to look, I found

(Cont.)

(Cont.)

that if I stepped aside from fear, I could find the strength in myself that I needed to deal with progressive vision loss.

Rather than seeing myself as different from those who do not have physical challenges, I began to realize how similar I am to everyone else in the world, whether they have diabetes or not. Each of us struggles in one way or another. Each of us laughs. Each of us cries. And all of us strive and stretch to live life to the fullest. I am no different in that respect from any other person.

Diabetes has taken things away from me, and it would be dishonest to deny the frustration I experience from living with inconvenience. But diabetes has also given. It has taught me things I could not have learned through any other means. When the illusion of good health was stripped away, I was left with introspection, and I now have the ability to see within myself.

When I began to lose my sight, a sense we all prize as essential, I was forced to find other resources, those that like deep beneath physical senses. There are talents, gifts, and skills that are just as essential as senses and they are beyond the physical reaches of diabetes.

Because what I thought would never happen is beginning to happen, I have learned precisely how much is possible in my life. I have developed a deeper sense of my own strength and a greater sense of inner peace. Each new challenge I overcome and each new obstacle I face proves that not only can I survive this disease, but that I can thrive.

At times, I have thought of diabetes as my most hated obstacle. But through all the anger, tears, and challenges, it has often proved to be my greatest asset; for, not only has it enabled me to reach essential parts of who I am, but it has given me the ability to touch who I wish to be.

—*Joan Wolf, Minneapolis, Minnesota*

delicate operation to remove hemorrhages and scar tissue, stop bleeding, replace some of the vitreous (the clear fluid within the eye) with a salt solution, and sometimes repair the detached retina. Laser therapy and vitrectomy should be performed by an ophthalmologist who specializes in retinal disease and who is experienced in these procedures in people with diabetes.

New ways to prevent and slow the development of retinopathy are being actively investigated. Researchers are looking into the effects of keeping blood glucose levels as near normal as possible in type I and type II diabetes. The use of naturally occurring substances called prostaglandins to control dilation and constriction of retinal blood vessels and other drugs is being studied.

Because the changes that occur with retinopathy may happen without any noticeable symptoms, regular eye exams are crucial for early detection and treatment.

CARDIOVASCULAR DISEASE

Good cardiovascular health deserves to be a priority for everyone. Taking care of your heart and the complex network of blood vessels in your body can reduce your chances of stroke, heart attack, and amputation, diabetes or no diabetes. However, the fact is that people with type II diabetes must work much harder than people without diabetes to ensure their cardiovascular health. The risk factors for cardiovascular disease seem to go hand in hand with type II diabetes: obesity, increased levels of blood fats, high blood levels of glucose and insulin, and high blood pressure. Cardiovascular disease is the most common cause of death in people with type II diabetes.

What is cardiovascular disease? It can go by many different names, but they all describe problems with the heart and circulatory system. The flow of blood through the body provides all the oxygen and other substances needed to have the energy to run your body. When blood flow is cut off, cells can die. Cigarette smoking, which causes the narrowing of blood vessels over time, is a major risk factor for cardiovascular disease. Blood flow can be cut off when blood vessels become clogged; this is arteriosclerosis, sometimes called hardening of the arteries. Vessels can become clogged by several ways: excess blood lipids (cholesterol and triglycerides) can cling to the vessel walls; the proteins carrying cholesterol and other blood fats can become covered with extra glucose, making them "sticky"; and there can be abnormalities in the blood-clotting mechanism.

Some arteries become clogged more commonly than others. One of these is the coronary artery, which supplies blood to the heart itself. A temporary slowdown in the blood supply to the heart leads to the pain of angina; a complete, longer-lasting stoppage of blood flow is described as a crushing pressure on the chest or a heart "attack." A blockage of any of the blood vessels supplying the brain is known as a stroke. Peripheral arterial disease, which is common in type II diabetes of long standing, usually involves leg blood vessels and can result in periods of intense pain with walking, often in the calves (intermittent claudication).

An all too common disability associated with diabetes is amputation. Of the diabetes complications involving the circulatory system, amputation is the easiest to avoid! Why does amputation still occur? When peripheral arterial disease, causing poor circulation in the extremities, occurs with the loss of sensation because of peripheral neuropathy, you have a pre-scription for trouble. It is possible to suffer foot damage without knowing it. Stepping on a pin can start a foot ulcer (open sore) that becomes infected. Trying to get rid of a feeling of coldness in the feet can lead to inadvertently scalding them with hot water or a heating pad. Impaired circulation also causes the healing process to be slowed down or impaired. Home surgery for foot problems can lead to even worse problems. (A podiatrist will warn you against **any** home surgery.) Failing to check your feet every day and letting these problems go without getting immediate medical attention can be disastrous.

Treatment

Treatments for cardiovascular disease are many. Some that are right for you could be as obvious as stabilizing blood glucose levels, losing weight, getting aerobic exercise, cutting down on fats in the diet. Most important, stop smoking, if you do. This program is the therapy of choice for all types of cardiovascular disease. Without question, however, quitting smoking is the one most guaranteed to add years of life.

There are minor surgical procedures that can open blocked blood vessels effectively. Balloon angioplasty, in which a small balloon is inflated to push open the blockage, and atherectomy, where blockage in a vessel is opened by boring a hole through it, require little "down" time. The use of laser light is a new approach to melt away blockages.

More serious surgery is arterial bypass surgery. This involves replacing a blocked artery with a blood vessel taken from another part of the body. The new artery or vein is obtained from the chest wall or leg (it must be large) and sewn above and below the blockage. Blood then flows around the blockage.

Intermittent claudication is usually treated with exercise and/ or drug therapy. The appearance of foot ulcers or infection may require surgery. In cases of stroke, normalization of blood glucose, blood pressure, and blood lipid levels, rehabilitation therapy, and medication aimed at correcting abnormal clotting mechanisms are the typical treatments; occasionally surgery is needed. Treatment of angina is aimed at reducing the amount of oxygen the heart tissue requires and increasing the amount of oxygen going to the heart. Besides the obvious solutions of quitting smoking, getting more exercise, normalizing blood pressure, and losing weight, medications such as nitrates, beta-adrenergic blockers, and calcium-channel blockers may be used. Surgery may be needed when these are not sufficient or on an urgent basis when the death of heart tissue is likely to occur.

Foot ulcers and other things that concern you about your feet should always be seen by your primary care physician or podiatrist immediately. Letting things go is the fastest way to wind up off your feet.

INFECTIONS

It probably won't surprise you to find out that infections are a common complication of diabetes. High blood glucose levels alter many body functions, among them the way the immune system works. Cells that attack invading bacteria and fungi become less effective and poor circulation prevents them from reaching the infection site or their killing activity is impaired.

On top of this, excess glucose supplies the food to fuel the invaders, especially a fungus like yeast.

Other diabetes complications add to the decreased ability to ward off infection. Autonomic neuropathy of the bladder can cause unawareness that the bladder is full or incomplete emptying—both of which can lead to urinary tract infection. Peripheral neuropathy can result in lost sensation in the extremities; without pain to warn of injury, an infection has time to take hold. Slowed or blocked blood flow prevents oxygen and infection-fighting white blood cells from reaching their target. Bacterial waste products, such as gas, can build up in tissues and do their own damage.

It's difficult to predict where an infection might occur. The skin and gums surrounding the teeth are especially vulnerable. Some women are prone to recurrent vaginal infections by the fungus *Candida* because of high glucose levels in this moist environment. People with diabetes also tend to have more hard-to-heal respiratory ailments than people without diabetes. Bacterial gangrene can also occur. This is an infection, usually found in a leg or foot, that starts with an opening in the skin and ends up killing the tissue. It takes hold very quickly if left untreated.

Treatment

All infections are helped by decreasing blood glucose levels toward normal. Bacterial and fungal infections can be treated with intravenous, oral, or topical medications. The best results are obtained when infections are noticed and treated early. Sometimes removal of layers of skin (debridement), drainage of pus, and immobilization are necessary in treating deep foot infections; the worst care scenario leads to amputation. Vaginal candidiasis can be treated with nonprescription creams; make sure your primary care physician diagnoses candidiasis before you begin treatment.

COEXISTING HEALTH CONCERNS

Because of the nature of type II diabetes, chances are that diabetes is not your only health concern. Many people diagnosed with type II diabetes also suffer from hypertension, arthritis, or high levels of blood lipids. You may attribute these problems to "getting old," and feeling this way may be somewhat realistic.

Coexisting health problems can also threaten your good diabetes control. Mixing medications can be dangerous and have unexpected side effects. This is why good communication with and among the members of your health-care team is crucial. Each member should know what medications you are taking.

Arthritis

There are several types of arthritis.

- The most common is degenerative joint disease. Anyone who lives long enough will probably have some form of this type of arthritis. It results from wear and tear on joints and weight bearing, which lead to stiffness and pain.

- Rheumatoid arthritis is a crippling disease indicated by red, swollen, and extremely painful joints. This arthritis is thought to be caused by an immune system attack on innocent cells in the body.

- Gout is a rare and extremely painful form of arthritis that is more common in people with diabetes than people without diabetes. High blood levels of uric acid form crystals in the joints, most commonly the big toe. The use of diuretics to control high blood pressure can contribute to uric acid formation. This is the only arthritis treated by dietary changes: eating animal organs such as liver and kidneys can lead to uric acid buildup. Specific drugs are also available to control uric acid levels.

If you suffer from arthritis, you need to be alert to the possibility that your arthritis medications may affect your blood glucose control or interact with your oral diabetes medications. Interactions with any medications, prescription or over-the-counter, need to be carefully managed by your primary care physician. Large doses of aspirin, for example, can lower blood glucose and thereby increase the potency of oral diabetes medications. Phenacetin and nonsteroidal anti-inflammatory drugs can harm the kidneys. Be sure to inform any specialist you might consult about arthritis that you have diabetes and about the other medications you take.

SOME DRUGS THAT CAN AFFECT BLOOD GLUCOSE LEVELS

Generic Name	Common Brand Names	Effect on Blood Glucose Level	Interacts With Oral Diabetes Medication?	Common Uses
Alcohol	As an ingredient in many prescription or over-the-counter medications	Lowers	Yes	Carries the active ingredient in the drug into the metabolism
Aspirin	Sold under many brand names	May lower if taken in large doses	Yes	Treating general pain or fever; treating arthritis
Beta-adrenergic blockers	Indural, Sectral, Tenormin, Lopressor, Corgard, Visken, Blocadren	Raises* or may mask hypoglycemia	Yes	Treating hypertension, angina, unsteady heartbeat, overactive thyroid, and other ailments
Chloramphenicol	Chloromycetin	Lowers†	Yes	Treating bacterial infections
Clofibrate	Atromid-S	Lowers†	Yes	Treating high cholesterol and triglyceride levels
Corticosteroids	Prednisone, Decadron, Kenalog, Cortisone	Raises	Yes	Treating inflammation, redness, and swelling in various disorders
Coumarin anticoagulants	Dicumarol	Lowers†	Yes	Preventing blood clots
Diazoxide	Hyperstat, Proglycem	Raises	Yes	Treating low blood glucose caused by pancreatic tumors; sometimes used for treating hypertension
Diuretics	Diuril, Hydro-DIURIL, Esidrix, Diamox, Lasix	Raises	Yes	Relieving fluid buildup by increasing volume of urine
Epinephrine or adrenaline	Adrenalin	Raises	Yes	Reviving heartbeat; treating severe allergic reactions
Epinephrine-like drugs (decogestants, cold products)	Pseudoephedrine, phenylpropanolamine, phenylephrine	Raise	Yes	Treating runny noses, allergies, colds

(Cont.)

(Cont.)

Generic Name	Common Brand Names	Effect on Blood Glucose Level	Interacts With Oral Diabetes Medication?	Common Uses
Estrogens, birth control pills	Sold under many brand names	May raise	No	Preventing pregnancy; lessening the effects of menopause
Fenfluramine	Pondimin	Lowers	No	Suppressing appetite
Lithium carbonate	Eskalith, Lithane	Raises	No	Treating manic depressive illness
Methyldopa	Aldomet	Lowers[†]	Yes	Treating high blood pressure
Monoamine oxidase (MAO) inhibitors	Parnate, Nardil, Eutonyl	Lowers	Yes	Treating severe depression
Nicotine transdermal patch	Nicoderm, Habitrol, Prostep	Lowers[‡]	No	Assisting in smoking cessation
Nicotinic acid, niacin	Nicolar, Nicobid	Raises	No	Treating nutrition deficiency; treating high cholesterol levels
Phenobarbital	Sold under many brand names	Raises[†]	Yes	Sedating; treating epilepsy
Phenytoin	Dilantin	Raises	Yes	Treating epilepsy and other nervous system disorders
Rifampin	Rifadin	Raises[†]	Yes	Treating tuberculosis
Sulfa drugs	Gantrisin, Septra, Bactrim	Lowers[†]	Yes	Treating bacterial infections
Thyroid preparations, desiccated thyroid		Raises	No	Treating thyroid deficiency

[*]*Beta-adrenergic blockers can raise blood glucose levels in most people with type II, but in some, they may lower blood glucose levels.*

[†]*These drugs raise or lower blood glucose only when used in combination with oral diabetes medications.*

[‡]*In general, quitting smoking lowers that amount of insulin you need. If you quit smoking and use the nicotine transdermal patch, be aware that your blood glucose level may drop and you may need to consult your physician about insulin adjustment.*

Hypertension

It is estimated that hypertension affects 20 percent of the adult population in the United States. Genetic background, body weight, and salt intake all play a role in the development of high blood pressure. Blacks have a much higher rate of hypertension than whites. But the greatest risk factor for developing hypertension is having type II diabetes: in one study, 60 percent of people who had type II diabetes more than 10 years also had high blood pressure.

If you have hypertension, it is extremely important to treat it effectively. Alone, it can do considerable damage to small blood vessels and capillaries, especially in the eyes and kidneys. Add type II diabetes, and the risk of damaging these delicate tissues or aggravating cardiovascular disease increases dramatically.

Treatment for hypertension usually starts with diet (low in sodium; low in fat if weight loss is needed) and exercise. Quitting smoking and limiting alcohol use are also important treatments. There are several kinds of oral medication for hypertension— diuretics, beta-adrenergic blockers, central adrenergic inhibitors, alpha-1 blockers, angiotensin-converting enzyme inhibitors, calcium-channel blockers, and vasodilators. One of these medications or a combination will be right for you. Be aware that some of these medications can throw your blood glucose levels out of balance and interact with your oral diabetes medication to produce side effects. Others can affect cholesterol and triglyceride levels. Anytime you try a new medication, look for reactions and discuss them with your physician. For more about blood pressure, see Chapter 3.

Blood Lipid Abnormalities

Type II diabetes, obesity, and abnormal blood fat profiles often go together. Researchers are questioning whether blood lipid abnormalities may contribute to obesity and, ultimately, type II diabetes. However, note that if hyperlipidemia (high levels of blood fats) is severe or if it occurs in other family members, even those without diabetes, this may indicate a lipid disorder unrelated to diabetes that also needs to be evaluated and treated.

Treatment for high levels of LDL cholesterol (the "bad" kind; see Chapter 3) and triglycerides usually means losing weight, improving blood glucose levels, increasing activity, and eating a low-fat high-fiber diet. All of these will be beneficial to your type II diabetes. A visit to a dietitian will assist you in making major changes in your eating habits.

If medications are needed, you must watch for changes in your blood glucose levels; you may have to self-monitor your blood glucose more times each day. Some medications can interfere with the breakdown, absorption, and removal of others. Many different types of medications are used to treat high blood lipid levels. Side effects are common; you should report anything unusual to your primary care physician.

Lifestyle
Considerations

CHAPTER 6

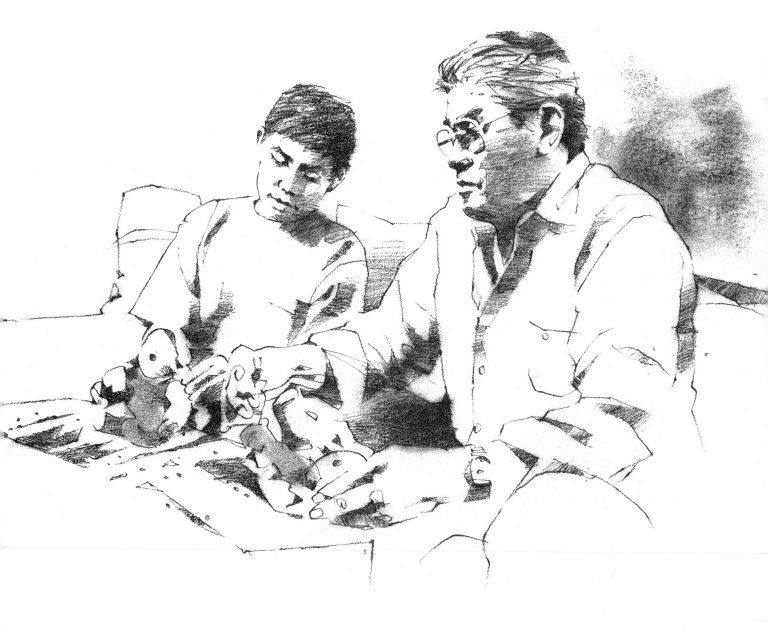

CAREERS AND EMPLOYMENT

Having diabetes doesn't have to affect your choice of employment or your performance at work. As long as you plan ahead, you will be able to work and control your diabetes. Because you need to eat regularly, it may be best for you to bring your own lunch and snacks. You may want to explain to your employers and colleagues how your condition affects your lifestyle. Emphasize that you must have regular hours with scheduled breaks for exercise and snacks.

Generally, you have the same needs as other people. To stay well, you must take good care of yourself, eat right, exercise regularly, have regular medical checkups, and receive appropriate and competent treatment for your medical condition.

People With Diabetes Are Desirable Workers

Living with diabetes takes diligence and self-discipline. People who have the disease are responsible for managing their glucose levels. The self-discipline required to do this usually leads to excellent work habits. Feel good about yourself and be sure to stress to your employer that "having diabetes can make you an even better employee."

Tips for Job Hunting

If you decide you need to find another career, there are many open to you. Some, however, because they have regular hours may be more desirable. Jobs that require that you work a variety of shifts can a bit more difficult to manage.

Here are a few tips to remember when you are job hunting.

- Don't regard your diabetes as a defect. Likewise, don't ask for special treatment because of it. It's best to be treated the same as any new employee.

- Prepare ahead of time by knowing your rights. For instance, employers usually are not permitted to ask questions about your health before deciding whether to hire you. Once they've offered you the job, however, they can ask health-related questions as part of the employment physical examination.

- If you decide to disclose your diabetes during your interview or your physical exam, then present a truthful picture of your condition and your control. You may want to refer to any awards you received in previous jobs or point out how few sick days you've ever taken. If you exercise regularly to stay fit, you may want to describe your routine.

■ Keep written notes about your job search at every step. If you are rejected for a position, ask for a written explanation. Keep copies of the job announcement and your job application. Make notes of your conversations and meetings with prospective employers, including dates, times, places, with whom you met, and the subjects discussed.

■ Be the best employee you can be. Arrive on time and don't call in sick unless it's absolutely necessary. Be honest with your employer about why you're absent. This way he or she will know it wasn't your diabetes that kept you from being at work.

The Employment Physical

If you have to take an employment physical, here are some suggestions for putting your best foot forward.

■ Don't change your treatment plan immediately before the examination. Changes in routine can affect control of your diabetes.

■ Remember that the company's doctor may not be a specialist in diabetes care. You may want to point out the steps you take to maintain control of your diabetes. Also, the doctor may not be aware of employment law and the legal protections that apply to people with a "hidden" disability, such as diabetes.

On the Job

Whether you inform your employer about your diabetes is completely up to you. Being open about your diabetes can educate others and reduce the perception that people with diabetes are somehow different. If you take insulin, it is useful for your coworkers to know how to recognize or even treat hypoglycemia.

Also, if something happens that requires you to make changes in your work schedule, your employer may understand

139

your need better and may feel that your openness was a sign of responsibility rather than a sign that you were hiding something. Always explain that as long as you take good care of yourself—by watching what you eat and getting enough exercise—you will be able to do your job.

Discrimination

Here are some suggestions for handling diabetes-related problems that occur on the job.

- Know what laws protect you. You may be covered by federal, state, or local laws and regulations. Your ADA Affiliate should have information on these laws.

- Try solving the problem by talking directly with your employer. American Diabetes Association materials may help, such as the pamphlet *A Word to Employers*.

- Enlist the help of your union or employee group.

- Consider seeing an attorney. With a telephone call or letter, an attorney may be able to resolve things quickly and amicably, making a lawsuit unnecessary. Your ADA Affiliate may have a list of attorneys interested in diabetes-related job discrimination.

- Continue to do the best job you can even while you are considering legal action. It is important to show that you care about your job and plan to keep it.

- Keep self-monitoring records in case you need to demonstrate your ability to maintain good control of your diabetes.

- See your primary care physician regularly. Your physician can be your strongest advocate, and you may want him or her to corroborate your health and your control of diabetes.

- If you are asked to leave, look for other work. If your case goes to court, the court may look for indications of your desire and ability to work.

Remedies

If you have been unfairly or wrongfully discharged, you may want to seek monetary compensation in the form of back pay, which is the sum of wages that you've lost. Or you may seek front pay, the amount of earnings that you would have enjoyed in the future but that were lost as a result of the damage done to your ability to earn a livelihood by being fired. You may also seek monetary compensation for emotional distress.

Alternatively, you may want to seek injunctive relief, resulting in your being reinstated to your position and/or benefits, such as seniority, vacation or retirement plan, or even a promotion if you would have otherwise received it but for the discrimination action you suffered.

Americans With Disabilities Act

When the Americans With Disabilities Act was enacted into federal law in 1990, it ensured equal opportunity for individuals with disabilities.

Under this law, diabetes is legally considered a disability. It defines a person with a disability as anyone who

- Has a physical or mental impairment that substantially limits one or more major life activities.

- Has a record of such an impairment.

- Is regarded as having such impairment.

141

GRAND CANYON SWEET

As we climbed into our car for the 10-minute drive to the trailhead, I cried, both from joy and from anticipation. Fifteen months before, just diagnosed with type II diabetes, my middle-aged, overweight self had trouble walking briskly one whole turn around the quarter-mile track at our local high school. Now I dared to tackle the Grand Canyon.

Having read up on the Canyon before our trip, I knew it could be treacherous, as well as enchanting. Aerobic fitness was essential for walking and hiking safely through its changing elevations.

Could I make it? I had my doubts. After all, I had been sedentary. I had been through yo-yo weight gains and losses until diabetes made me realize I had to exercise and control my eating now—no more maybes or tomorrows.

(Cont.)

(Cont.)

But then again, I had reason to be confident. Since beginning my diabetic diet, I had lost 30 pounds and perhaps more importantly, had exercised faithfully. By walking and using a cross-country ski machine, I had maintained a regimen of aerobic workouts at least four times a week.

My husband and I had decided to make our first day at the Canyon a trial of our abilities (even he wasn't sure of his capabilities in a strange environment). We had done some hiking and camping in the Appalachian Mountains, but we had never experienced high-altitude hiking or desert conditions, both of which occur within the Grand Canyon.

We would first try a short, yet strenuous hike, 3 miles round trip, with a 1,500-foot elevation change. As promised in our guidebook, we got marvelous views, and we completed the hike in less time than the three hours.

We spent the next day exploring the rim by foot and shuttle bus.

By our third day, we were ready to try the 12-mile round-trip hike along Bright Angel Trail, a path first carved by Indians, now used by hikers and mules trains to travel to and from the Colorado River.

Our route would take us 9 miles down, then 3,200 feet up to Indian Gardens where we'd find water and shade. Then we'd have a 3-mile side trip to get a bird's-eye view of the Colorado River. The side trip meant walking under a relentless sun through the desert where the temperature was 100 degrees.

By the end of the day, the climb back to the rim had challenged my physical endurance to the limit: I had worked aerobically for four and a half hours. I ended my adventure exhausted and exhilarated. I would never ask to have diabetes, but since I do have it, I'm glad it motivated me to get into shape. I had not known how emotionally uplifting fitness can be.

—*Tullia Limarzi, New York, New York*

Under this law, if you work for a private employer who has 25 or more employees (this will change to 15 employees in 1994) and you feel you have been discriminated against due to your disability, you have the right to file a complaint with the appropriate government agency and have the situation corrected.

The new law will not give you preference if you are competing with someone equally qualified. Just as in any employment situation, employers have the option of choosing whomever they feel can best perform the job. However, an employer will run into problems if he or she hires someone less qualified, while refusing employment to a better-qualified person who happens to have diabetes or any other disability.

PREGNANCY AND BIRTH CONTROL

Being pregnant and having a baby can be an awesome enough experience without your having additional concerns about your diabetes. So plan the safest and most appropriate time to have a child. Maintain excellent blood glucose control **before** you become pregnant. Once you make the decision to try to conceive, you should strive for normal blood glucose levels. Good diabetes management is important both before and during pregnancy: it reduces the chances of giving birth to an infant with birth defects or other problems.

Of course, **planning** a pregnancy means that you are going to use some form of birth control until you are ready to have that baby. Which form of contraception you use is entirely up to you and your partner. The pill, diaphragm and cervical cap plus spermicidal jelly, sponge, and condom plus spermicidal foam are all good ways to prevent pregnancy. Consult your primary care physician and gynecologist about which method is best for you.

The Pill

For women with diabetes, the pill may increase blood glucose levels and is suspected of increasing the risk of complications. The short-term risks (during the first year or two of use) are slight, but scientists are not certain about the risks of using the pill for longer periods of time. If you develop high blood pressure while taking the pill, this could increase the risk that retinopathy or kidney disease will progress. In some individuals, the estrogen part of the pill raises blood fat levels. Because of these possibilities, you need to know whether you have any complications before you start using birth control pills.

Pregnancy and Diabetes Control

As stated above, it is very important to keep your blood glucose levels normal throughout pregnancy. To help keep yourself in excellent control when pregnant and give yourself the best chances for a healthy baby, you need to add an obstetrician with experience and interest in caring for women with diabetes to your health-care team.

Do I Need a Special Diet?

When you become pregnant, a special visit to your dietitian is in order to help you make any dietary changes you need to meet the demands of pregnancy. Three meals and three snacks a day are often the rule. Occasionally, a middle-of-the-night snack may be necessary to keep your metabolism normal.

Meal planning during pregnancy means making sure you gain enough weight over the nine months. A weight gain of 22 to 32 pounds over the nine-month period is normal. If you are overweight, your weight gain may be limited to 15 pounds. Your primary care provider or obstetrician will tell you how much weight you will can gain.

Check with your physician to see whether an occasional glass of wine or mug of beer is permissible. However, do not smoke or abuse drugs when pregnant. These may harm your baby seriously.

Should I Still Take My Medications?

Oral diabetes medications are not recommended for use during pregnancy. Options are to gain good enough control to do without the pills or to start treatment with insulin.

Because many medications can be harmful to your baby, don't take any medications unless they were prescribed for you to take **during** pregnancy or you have checked with your physician. Indeed, be sure to check with your physician even before you take over-the-counter medications.

Can I Still Exercise?

Exercise helps diabetes control. Pregnant women may be able to exercise by walking, swimming, and doing other kinds of aerobic exercise. Generally, you will be able to continue an exercise you were doing regularly before pregnancy. Your physician needs to approve of any exercise you want to do.

Will I Need Additional Insulin?

If your type II diabetes is controlled with diet only, you may need to begin taking insulin during pregnancy. If you are already taking insulin, you may have to increase the dosage. Some women require two or three times more insulin than usual during pregnancy, especially toward the end of pregnancy. This is normal and does not necessarily indicate that your diabetes control is sliding. Do not change your insulin dosage without advice from your primary care physician. After delivery, and if you breastfeed, after weaning, you will likely return to your prepregnancy diabetes treatment program.

Do I Need to Test My Blood Glucose Level?

You will need to test your blood glucose more often when you're pregnant. This will help your primary care physician properly adjust your insulin and diet to keep blood glucose levels normal.

Must I Make Special Arrangements for Delivering My Baby?

Your health-care team will decide the best time and way of delivery. Usually, delivery at a hospital is preferred because many babies born to women with diabetes are delivered by Cesarean section (C-section). A C-section is an operation in which a cut is made through the lower abdomen and uterus to remove the baby. If you have a C-section, you will need to stay in the hospital four to five days. It takes four to six weeks to fully recover.

Will My Baby Be Healthy?

With excellent diabetes control and expert care, the chances for a healthy baby are great and the risk of a problem is no greater than in a nondiabetic pregnancy.

Sometimes, however, the baby of a diabetic woman may be bigger and weigh more than normal. That is why C-sections are more common among diabetic women. If diabetes control has not been good, the baby also may have difficulty breathing; low blood glucose; low blood calcium; or jaundice, a yellowing of the skin. All of these conditions can be treated but are best prevented by keeping normal blood glucose levels throughout pregnancy.

The chances for birth defects are low if diabetes control is excellent during the first 12 weeks of pregnancy. To enhance your chances of giving birth to a healthy baby, get yourself in excellent diabetes control before pregnancy, keep your control excellent, and follow the advice of your health-care team.

Will Breastfeeding Pose Any Additional Problems?

Having diabetes need not prevent you from having a successful breastfeeding experience. As you might have guessed, the best way to avoid problems is to practice good diabetes control during the months you breastfeed your baby. You will probably find yourself hungrier and thirstier than normal.

Breastfeeding may affect your blood glucose control. You may have erratic blood glucose levels and an increase in insulin reactions. Or your diabetes may be easier to control, resulting in your being able to eat a little more and take less medication.

THE GREAT ESCAPE

When my kids are screaming at each other over whose turn it is to watch television and my wife is asking for my assistance in getting the house respectable for my mother's visit, I excuse myself to take my 6-mile run.

Exercise is a main component in controlling my diabetes. Forcing myself to run even when I don't want to is just part of the mental discipline that I have to maintain. Escaping from screaming kids and not having to clean a messy garage is just a lucky coincidence.

—*Robert A. Fellman, Nashville, Tennessee*

You probably will have to test your blood glucose level more often in the months that you breastfeed. You will need to take extra precautions and have some form of fast-acting sugar (see Chapter 3) close at hand so you can treat any insulin reactions. A good habit is to snack and drink a glass of water just before you start a breastfeeding session. You may have to change your medication regimen and meal plan. Don't make any of these changes without first consulting your primary care physician or endocrinologist.

Breastfeeding can be a wonderful experience for you and your baby. Think of the extra plus you are providing for your baby in terms of antibodies (protection against infection) and an "allergy-proof" formula that no canned formula can duplicate. And breastfeeding may provide the motivation you need to continue good blood glucose control. The good habits you cultivate during your pregnancy and while you breastfeed can last a lifetime—and so can the advantages of good blood glucose control.

DIABETES IN THE FAMILY

Diabetes is a family disease in more ways than one.

The fact that diabetes tends to occur in members of a family is old news. We also know that habits that lead to obesity, poor diet, and lack of exercise can be learned in a family. But in addition, research on families with type II diabetes has revealed evidence that genetic susceptibility also plays a role.

The influence of genetics in the development of type II diabetes has been confirmed in studies of identical twins. Researchers found that the identical twin of a person who has type II diabetes goes on to develop type II diabetes with almost certainty. Research on the Pimas, American Indians who have the highest rate of type II diabetes of all Americans, has shown that families can be labeled as "insulin resistant" or "insulin sensitive." These studies suggest that certain families may be able to resist developing diabetes better than others.

You may or may not be able to determine whether your family has a tendancy to develop insulin resistance that is passed on in the genes. However, you may be able to guess whether obesity due to overeating and a sendentary lifestyle has contributed to insulin resistance. We know that a tendancy toward type II diabetes does not mean that insulin resistance cannot be reversed. Weight-loss and exercise programs have proved too successful to discount the power of behavior over genetic susceptibility.

Preventing Type II Diabetes

Are your children, siblings, or even parents at risk for type II diabetes? If a genetic component was at work to cause your type II diabetes, then the answer is yes. If your children have

147

followed your lead in developing obesity related to inactivity and poor eating habits, the answer is also yes.

How can you help your children and other relatives give themselves the best chance of not developing type II diabetes?

- Realize that your new eating habits are healthy for everyone. Don't isolate yourself because of your meal plan—prepare family meals that everyone can enjoy.

- Involve them in your education. Encourage them to visit your physician and dietitian with you.

- Make sure they have regular checkups with a primary care physician experienced and interested in diabetes. Early detection of insulin resistance or fat metabolism disorders may mean diabetes prevention.

- Ask your children to be your exercise partners. Set goals together and help keep each other motivated.

- Encourage them to fight the "fat monster." Set a good example!

The diagnosis of type II diabetes in one family member often means drastic changes in lifestyle and food and exercise habits for the entire family. Developing and maintaining good eating and exercise habits could mean the difference between life with diabetes and life without it.

ALCOHOL USE

There is no evidence that an **occasional mealtime drink** is harmful to people with diabetes in good control. Contrary to common belief, small amounts of alcohol close to or with a meal produce little change in the blood glucose levels of people with diabetes.

Heavy drinking and dependency on alcohol, however, is dangerous for anyone. Mixing alcohol and prescription or over-the-counter medications can be very dangerous.

Alcoholic beverages supply calories but little or no nutrients. If you are dieting to lose weight or trying to keep to your diet plan, alcohol can disrupt your diet control. You may want to try alcohol-free beer and wine. Just remember, these drinks are not calorie free!

Here are some precautions to take if you're going to have alcoholic drinks.

- Consult your physician to find out how much, if any, drinking is safe for you. Because large amounts of alcohol can be toxic to organs, you will be advised not to drink alcohol if you have gastritis (inflammation of the stomach), pancreatitis (inflammation of the pancreas), liver disease, certain forms of heart or kidney disease, or take particular medications.

- Avoid habitual heavy drinking or you may develop other medical problems. Heavy drinkers can develop a condition called hypertriglyceridemia (excessive levels of blood fats called triglycerides). Hypertriglyceridemia can cause abdominal pain, pancreatitis, and skin rashes. It may also contribute to hardening of the arteries and being overweight. At a minimum, heavy drinking will make blood glucose control more difficult.

- Do not drink on an empty stomach. It can exaggerate the blood glucose–lowering action of insulin or oral diabetes medications and interfere with the body's ability to produce its own glucose in response to falling blood glucose levels. Even a mild hypoglycemic reaction during drinking is of special concern to people with diabetes. First, the effects of a low blood glucose level on the brain may be worsened by the effects of alcohol. Second, alcohol on the breath may mislead people into thinking you are merely intoxicated. The treatment you need for hypoglycemia may then be delayed.

- If you are being treated with oral diabetes medications, do not drink unless you have sought and received approval from your physician. Alcohol can enhance the effects of some of these kinds of medications, even causing dizziness, flushing, and severe nausea. Eating usually helps to alleviate these sensations.

Which Drinks Are Best?

Choose drinks that are lower in alcohol and sugar. Very sweet dessert wines, such as port and liqueurs, have too much sugar (up to 50 percent) and alcohol (up to 30 percent). The simple sugar typically found in very sweet drinks enters the

149

ALCOHOLIC BEVERAGES AND MIXES

Beverage	Serving (ounces)	Alcohol (grams)	Carbohydrates (grams)	Calories	Exchanges for Calorie Control
Beer					
Regular	12	13	13	150	1 Starch, 2 Fat
Light	12	11	5	100	2 Fat,
Near beer	12	1.5	12	60	1 Starch
Distilled spirits, 80 proof (gin, rum vodka, whiskey, scotch)	1.5	14	Trace	100	2 Fat
Dry brandy, cognac	1	11	Trace	75	1.5 Fat
Table wine					
Dry white	4	11	Trace	80	2 Fat
Red or rosé	4	12	2	85	2 Fat
Sweet wine	4	12	5	105	⅓ Starch, 2 Fat
Light wine	4	6	1	50	1 Fat
Wine cooler	12	13	30	215	2 Fruit, 2 Fat
Dealcoholized wines	4	Trace	6–7	25–35	0.5 Fruit
Sparkling wines					
Champagne	4	12	4	100	2 Fat
Sweet kosher wine	4	12	12	132	1 Starch, 2 Fat
Appetizer/ dessert wines					
Sherry	2	9	2	74	1.5 Fat
Sweet sherry, port, muscatel	2	9	7	90	0.5 Starch, 1.5 Fat
Cordias, liqueurs	1.5	13	18	160	1 Starch, 2 Fat
Vermouth					
Dry	3	13	4	105	2 Fat
Sweet	3	13	14	140	1 Starch, 2 Fat
Cocktails					
Bloody Mary	5	14	5	116	1 Vegetable, 2 Fat
Daiquiri	2	14	2	111	2 Fat
Manhattan	2	17	2	178	2.5 Fat
Martini	2.5	22	Trace	156	3.5 Fat
Old Fashioned	4	26	Trace	180	4 Fat
Tom Collins	7.5	16	3	120	2.5 Fat

(Cont.)

(*Cont.*) Mixes					
Mineral water	Any	0	0	0	Free
Sugar-free tonic	Any	0	0	0	Free
Club soda	Any	0	0	0	Free
Diet soda	Any	0	0	0	Free
Tomato juice	4	0	5	25	1 Vegetable
Bloody Mary mix	4	0	5	25	1 Vegetable
Orange juice	4	0	15	60	1 Fruit
Grapefruit juice	4	0	15	60	1 Fruit
Pineapple juice	4	0	15	60	1 Fruit

bloodstream more rapidly than complex carbohydrate and can cause a sharp rise in blood glucose. If you use mixers in your drinks, the best choices are ones that are low in sugar or sugar free, such as diet soft drinks, diet tonic, club soda, seltzer, or water.

Light beer and dry wines are recommended also, because they have less alcohol and less carbohydrates, and therefore, fewer calories. Examples of dry white wines are Chablis, dry chenin blanc, chardonnay, French Colombard, dry sauterne, dry sauvignon blanc, white burgundy, and dry Riesling. Some dry red wines include burgundy, cabernet sauvignon, claret, gamay Beaujolais, merlot, Pinot noir, and zinfandel. Consider drinking dry rose, dry champagne, and dry sherry.

Working Alcohol Into Your Meal Plan

If, in consultation with your health-care team, it is agreed that occasional mealtime drinking is safe for you, you can construct a list of calories and/or exchanges for your favorite drinks. Be sure to subtract those drinks from your day's meal plan.

Be sure to obtain specific information about the wines you drink most often. Wines can differ in alcohol and sugar content from winery to winery. Most wine labels include the percentage of alcohol, and some labels also list the amount of residual sugar. If the wine is not dry or the label does not have the information you need, consider writing to the winery or talk to the store owner. Knowledgeable wine merchants can be very helpful in providing you information about the characteristics of various wines.

Calories and Exchanges

It's best if alcohol does not contribute more than six percent of the day's total calories. To make your alcoholic drinks last longer, consider mixing wine with sparkling water, club soda, or diet soda to make "spritzer"; try unusual flavors of diet seltzers. Virgin Marys (without any alcohol) may be as satisfying as Bloody Marys.

Because alcoholic drinks are generally calculated as Fat exchanges, divide the calories in the drink by 45 (the number of calories in 1 Fat exchange). A can of light beer, which has approximately 97 calories, for example, would contain two Fat exchanges. So if you consume a can of light beer, you would have to subtract two Fat exchanges from your meal plan. Occasionally, you may prefer to exchange a bread or meat for an alcoholic drink. It's okay as long as you are sure that the rest of your diet is nutritionally sound.

As an alternative, many nutritionists calculate alcoholic beverages that contain carbohydrate—notably regular beer and sweet wines—in terms of Fat and Starch/Bread. The alcohol is exchanged for Fat, and the carbohydrate is exchanged for Starch/Bread.

If you use calorie-containing mixers, use an appropriate exchange group for substitution. For example, for orange juice, omit the necessary number of Fruit exchanges; for tomato juice, subtract Vegetable exchanges; and for cream, use Fat exchanges.

Thus, a Bloody Mary, made with a jigger of vodka and 3/4 cup (6 ounces) of tomato juice, would have approximately 142 calories (107 from the 1 1/2 ounces of alcohol plus 35 from the juice). This is equivalent to about 2 Fat exchanges from the vodka and 1 vegetable exchange from the tomato juice.

Cooking With Alcohol

When alcohol is heated in cooking, either over direct heat or in the oven, most of it evaporates. This leaves few calories. Alcohol as wine, brandy, or sherry is a good way to add flavor to foods you cook, and the calories do not need to be calculated in your meal plan.

General Guidelines for Alcohol Use

Drinking alcohol may weaken your resolve to follow your meal plan. Also, drinking by someone who is fasting or on a very-low-calorie diet may lead to hypoglycemia. This could be a serious problem if you are taking oral diabetes medications or insulin. Try to build these habits

- Before you start drinking, decide how much you will eat and drink.
- Put less alcohol in your drink.
- Drink slowly. Make one drink last.
- Don't drink without eating, too.
- Don't drink and drive.
- Talk to your primary care physician about how alcohol may affect any medications you may be taking.

Remember, alcohol is a drug. It can damage your body if you drink too much. To make alcohol a part of your meal plan, you need good judgment, and you should have your diabetes in good control.

DRUGS AND TOBACCO

Certain drugs raise your blood glucose, others lower it. Learning how legal and illegal drugs affect your diabetes control will help you avoid problems.

Tobacco

Smoking tobacco is especially dangerous for people with diabetes, who are at risk for heart disease and blood vessel disease. Smoking increases that risk.

Here are a few tips to help you quit smoking cigarettes, courtesy of the National Cancer Institute.

- Switch to a brand you don't like.
- Buy cigarettes lower in tar and nicotine.
- Put your packs in a different pocket or purse compartment so they won't be so easy to reach for.
- Target a final quitting date, then work toward it.
- Each day decide how many cigarettes you will smoke.
- Postpone your first cigarette for an hour or two, and try smoking only half a cigarette.

- Find a healthy habit, such as a quick walk after a meal, to replace smoking.
- Avoid situations that you associate with smoking until your resolve is strong.
- Talk to your physician about aids that assist smoking cessation.

Marijuana

Marijuana increases your appetite, making it more difficult to keep to your diet. If you eat more than you planned, your blood glucose may rise too high.

Cocaine

This drug raises your blood glucose level and changes your eating habits. It affects your moods. It can raise blood pressure or cause heart irregularities suddenly. Heavy use leads to atherosclerosis; the risk for this circulatory disease is already high for people with diabetes. Your chance of having a heart attack is multiplied.

Caffeine

Caffeine is found in coffee, tea, chocolate, and many soft drinks. It could raise your blood glucose level a small amount. Other side effects include not being able to sleep, shaking, and increased blood pressure and heart rate. You could confuse your reaction to caffeine as hypoglycemia.

Appetite Suppressants

Your doctor may prescribe these pills to help you lose weight. They may satisfy your hunger, so you won't eat. Be aware, however, that your blood glucose may fall and some cause jitteriness, heart palpitations, and loss of sleep.

Depressants

Sleeping pills and tranquilizers are depressants. Your doctor may prescribe them to help you sleep or to calm you down. These drugs will slow down your breathing and may hide symptoms of hypoglycemia.

TRAVEL

For a person with diabetes, the first rule of travel is this: You can go anywhere and do almost anything. It just takes a little advanced planning to handle your diabetes.

How you prepare will depend on your travel plans. Will you be traveling by plane, train, car, bicycle, boat, or a combination? Will you be crossing time zones? Plan ahead before you leave.

- For a lengthy trip, have a medical exam to make sure your diabetes is in control.

GOING PUBLIC

Former United States ambassador to France Joe M. Rodgers was diagnosed with type II diabetes when in his early 50s. He controls his diabetes through diet, exercise, and insulin. He is among the minority of people with type II diabetes who use insulin to help control their diabetes. Joe takes two insulin shots a day, and he exercises on a treadmill several times a week, making sure his workouts are long enough to get aerobic benefits from them.

"You can't use excuses like, 'Hey, I can't do my exercises because I'm traveling'...Don't get me wrong—I'm not perfect at exercising regularly—but I do try."

Joe learned first-hand to be extra careful when traveling. While on a trip to the Bahamas and running low on insulin, he decided to use some he'd left in his briefcase. "It must have been affected by the heat," he recalls, because the insulin had no effect on him. A few days later, he found himself in the hospital—doctors, however, had misinterpreted his symptoms as those of a heart attack. This episode taught him an important lesson: never take diabetes lightly.

Joe volunteers for the American Diabetes Association's National Advisory Council. Rodgers considers vital the council's work in raising money. In his eyes, raising funds is directly connected to research, and research is crucial to finding a cure. "Money can help do something about this disease," he says with conviction.

Joe is also concerned with the stigma that some people suffer because they have diabetes. "I'd hate for people who have diabetes to be afraid that others would know," he says. "Diabetes is a disease, not a stigma."

- Get a letter from your doctor saying that you have diabetes. Be sure the letter includes a statement that you must use oral diabetes medications or insulin and syringes and a list of other medications. Include any allergies, as well as food and medication sensitivities you may have.

- Get a prescription from your doctor for insulin or oral diabetes pills. In the United States, prescription rules may be different from state to state. And the laws may be very different in other countries. Don't risk being without insulin, syringes, or oral medications.

- Get a list of ADA Affiliates or chapters if you're traveling in the United States or look them up in the local phone book white pages. If you're going overseas, write for a list of International Diabetes Federation groups (see Resources).

- Get immunization shots—if you need them—at least one month before you leave.

- Order a medical ID bracelet or necklace that indicates that you have diabetes (see Resources).

- If you're leaving the country, learn how to say "I have diabetes" and "Sugar or orange juice, please," in several appropriate languages so you can make yourself understood wherever you are.

- You may also want to request a list of English-speaking foreign doctors (see Resources). If an emergency occurs while traveling and you don't have such a list, contact the American Consulate, American Express, or local medical schools for a list of doctors.

- If you're flying, remember your option of requesting a special meal. If you give yourself insulin injections, do so just as your food is coming down the aisle to avoid unforeseen delays and hypoglycemia.

A Special Note About Insulin

Insulins sold abroad are frequently of different strengths than the U-100 used in the U.S. If you buy insulin abroad and if it is a different strength (U-40 or U-80), you must buy new syringes to match the new insulin to avoid dosing errors. If you use U-100 syringes for U-40 or U-80 insulin, you will be taking much less insulin than was prescribed. Conversely, if you use U-100 insulin in a U-40 or U-80 syringe, you will be taking too much insulin.

Packing Tips

Pack twice as much medication and blood-testing equipment as needed, because it's always better to be on the safe side. Pack half in your carry-on luggage to keep your medications with you. Also, pack some extra food for yourself—cheese and crackers, juice, and fruit. Take comfortable shoes and clothes, sunglasses, suntan lotion, and whatever else will add to your comfort.

Ground Travel

You must make appropriate arrangements for storing medications. Insulin preparations contain bacteriostatic agents that make refrigeration unnecessary. Extreme temperatures (hot or cold), however, may cause a loss insulin potency. The major culprits to watch out for are the automobile glove compartment

CARRY-ON LUGGAGE CHECKLIST

Medications

    Insulins
    Syringes
    Oral diabetes medications
    Glucagon kit
    Glucose tablets or other sugar source
    Snacks, such as dried fruit or crackers
    Antinausea suppositories
    Other prescribed medications
    Antibiotic ointment

Blood-Testing Equipment

    Test strips
    Lancets
    Blood-sampling device and a spare
    Alcohol wipes (if used)
    Spare batteries for glucose meter
    Cotton or tissues

and trunk. Backpacks and cycle bags also can get quite hot in direct sunlight.

If you are traveling by car, insulin should be kept in an insulated container with ice or "blue ice" (but insulin must not be allowed to freeze), a cool damp cloth, or some other cooling agent. This is also necessary for antinausea suppositories, which can melt in extreme heat.

Crossing Time Zones

Here is a rule of thumb: eastward travel results in a shorter day; thus, if you inject insulin, less insulin may be needed. Conversely, westward travel, with its longer day, may require more insulin. If you have concerns about insulin adjustment while crossing time zones, take your round-trip airline flight schedule to your primary care physician or endocrinologist along with information on the time zone changes. Work out the appropriate adjustments in intermediate- or long-acting and short-acting insulins for travel days. These may depend on your meal schedule and plans for sleep or activity on arrival at your destination. Self-monitoring of blood glucose while traveling will always help you deal with any uncertainty.

Whether you travel eastward or westward, it's smart to watch what you eat and drink. Unusual foods may upset your stomach and hurt your diabetes control. Good diabetes control is as important on the road as at home.

EATING OUT

Today, more and more Americans are eating out at restaurants. If you plan in advance and choose foods wisely, the foods they offer can fit into your meal plan.

Restaurant owners are responding to their new health-conscious clientele. They're providing lower cholesterol, lower fat, lower sodium, and higher fiber food. All eating establishments offer sugar substitutes and diet beverages. Most serve fruit juice and decaffeinated coffee. Some have reduced-calorie salad dressings, low-fat or skim milk, and salt substitutes. It's easy to find salads, fish, seafood, vegetables, baked or broiled food, and whole-grain breads.

More restaurants are offering menus that list calories and nutritive values or provide the information on request. If you ask, chefs will usually create low-fat entrees made with low-cholesterol egg substitutes or lean cuts of meat. Some cooks will remove the skin from a chicken before cooking, omit extra butter on the dish, broil instead of fry, and serve sauces on the side. There are restaurants that will allow you to order small portions at reduced prices.

Table Tips

Not everyone with diabetes has the same meal plan or the same nutritional priorities. For some, cutting calories is most important, whereas others may need to avoid fat and eat high-fiber foods. Determine with your dietitian or primary care physician which of your personal goals are most important for you. Then you'll have some flexibility to deviate from your meal plan if the restaurant doesn't have exactly what you need—or if you're dining out for a special occasion.

If you regularly eat away from home, on business or for convenience, it's important to stick to your meal plan and timing as much as possible. You can do this more easily if you pick a restaurant that offers a wide variety of choices. Or, try to "brown-bag" your lunch to avoid eating out.

Order only what you need and want. Here are some ordering tips to follow:

- If you don't know the ingredients in a dish or the serving size, ask.

- Try to eat similar-sized portions to those you eat at home. If larger portions are served, put the excess in a "doggie bag" (before you start eating, if possible) or share portions with your dining partner.

- Eat slowly.

- Ask that added butter be left off the broiled fish or meat.

- Ask that sour cream or butter for the baked potato be put on the side (or left off altogether).

- Ask that no salt be added in preparing your food.

- Ask that sauces, gravy, and dressings be served on the side.

- Make sure the food you order isn't breaded and fried, which adds fat. If the food arrives breaded, peel off the outer coating.

160

MAKING HEALTHY CHOICES WHEN DINING OUT	
	Foods to Choose
Appetizers	Tomato juice, unsweetened fruit juice Clear broth, bouillon, consomme Raw (not marinated) vegetables; fresh fruit, unsweetened Fresh steamed seafood
Eggs	Poached, boiled
Salads	Tossed vegetable, lettuce, tomato, cucumber, onion Cottage cheese (as part of the Meat exchange allowance) Salads with low-calorie dressing, lemon juice, or vinegar
Breads	Whole-grain rolls or crackers, biscuits, or breads
Potatoes and substitutes	Baked, boiled, steamed potatoes Steamed rice or noodles
Fats	Diet margarine, low-calorie salad dressing, low-fat sour cream or yogurt (Remember to count the fat used on vegetables, if buttered in the kitchen, as 1 Fat exchange.)
Vegetables	Raw, stewed, steamed, boiled
Meat, poultry, and fish	Roasted, baked, or broiled Lean meats with fat trimmed Dishes without gravy or sauce
Desserts	Fresh fruit or fruit juice Ice cream (1/2–cup scoop = 1 Starch/Bread + 2 Fat exchanges)
Beverages	Coffee, tea (decaffeinated) Milk, according to your meal plan Diet soda

(Cont.)

(*Cont.*)

	Foods to Avoid
Appetizers	Cream soups, thick soups Sweetened juices Canned fruit cocktail Seafood cocktail (unless you plan to eat less meat later)
Eggs	Fried, creamed, and scrambled
Salads	Coleslaw and other salads with dressing (These are fine at home, but may have too much dressing in a restaurant.) Canned fruit or gelatin salads
Breads	Sweet rolls, coffee cake
Potatoes and substitutes	Fried, French fried, creamed, escalloped, au gratin
Fats	Gravy, fried foods, creamed foods
Vegetables	Creamed, escalloped, au gratin, in cheese sauce
Meats, poultry, and fish	Fatty, fried, and breaded foods Bacon and sausage Meats in cream sauce Stews and casserole-type dishes (It's better to eat these at home so you know what is in them.)
Desserts	Puddings, custard, pastry Sweetened fruits
Beverages	Chocolate milk, cocoa, milk shakes Regular soft drinks

- Read the menu creatively. For instance, order the fruit cup appetizer or the breakfast melon for your dinner dessert.

- Ask for substitutions, such as low-fat cottage cheese, baked potato, or even a double portion of a vegetable instead of french fries.

- Ask for low-calorie items, like salad dressings, even if they're not listed on the menu.

- Avoid alcohol. Substitute low-calorie or calorie-free beverages.

Some restaurants will better meet your special needs if you phone ahead. When you make the reservation, it's possible to ask that your food be prepared with vegetable oil, low-fat margarine, little salt, no extra sauce or butter, and broiled instead of fried.

Dining On Time

If you take oral diabetes medications or insulin, ordering the right foods isn't your only concern—the time of the meal is also important. Ask your meal companion to eat at your usual time. Make your plans so you won't be kept waiting for a table when you should be eating. Have reservations and be on time. Try to avoid the busiest hours at the restaurant so nothing goes wrong to keep you waiting. Ask whether "special" dishes will take extra time to be prepared and served.

If your lunch or dinner is going to be later than usual, eat a fruit or bread serving from that meal at your usual mealtime. If the dinner will be very late, you can have your bedtime snack at your dinner time, then eat the full dinner at the later hour. You may need to adjust your short-acting insulin doses to do this.

It's a good idea to let the restaurant manager know if you like the healthy choices you see on the menu. If you want more low-calorie, low-cholesterol choices should be on the menu, say so. Restaurants, like any business, offer what the customers want. And they only know what you want if you tell them.

The Fast Food Challenge

The key to making knowledgeable and healthy fast food choices is knowing exactly what you are ordering and to plan in advance. First, as always, eat a variety of foods in moderate portions, with about 30 percent of the daily calories from fat and no more than 3,000 milligrams of salt. Next, count calories. Keep within the guidelines your dietitian or physician has given you. It's also a great idea to count grams of fat. Your dietitian can tell you have many grams of fat per day can be eaten to stay within your total daily calorie intake. Many fast food restaurants will supply you with dietary information on their food if you ask.

Is it possible for fast food to be a healthy choice? The answer depends on what you order. It is possible to consume an entire day's worth of fat, salt, and calories in just one meal. The average calorie count of a fast food meal is 685, which is not outrageously high for a meal, but is usually too many calories for a snack. Words on a menu like "jumbo," "giant," or "deluxe" should signal caution. Larger serving sizes mean not only additional calories, but generally also more fat, cholesterol, and sodium.

It's important to make wise choices. If you have fast food for one meal, try to balance the rest of your day's food choices. Order items without toppings and rich sauces. Be suspicious of chicken, fish, and "light" items. Depending on their preparation, they are not always lower in fat, calories, and sodium.

Even though the changes being made in the fast food industry make it possible to select nutritionally sound food, the vast majority of fast food items remain high in fat. By knowing the nutritional value of fast food items, you can choose foods that will be consistent with your meal plan.

Several restaurants are offering special products lower in fat. For example, McDonald's has introduced its McLean hamburger, and Arby's has a variety of leaner "light" sandwich options. Hardee's offers several selections lower in fat, such as the grilled chicken sandwich. Wendy's also has a grilled chicken sandwich served on a multigrain bun. Burger King's BK Broiler is flame-broiled chicken served on an oat bran bun. And McDonald's has added a fat-free (but high in sugar) muffin to their breakfast options. However, Kentucky Fried Chicken advertises a skinless fried chicken that has hardly any less fat than the regular version.

FAST FOOD FACTS							
Product	Serving size	Calories	Carbo-hydrates (grams)	Protein (grams)	Fat (grams)	Sodium (milli-grams)	Exchanges
ARBY'S							
Junior Roast Beef	3 oz	218	22	12	8	345	1½ Starch/Bread, 1½ Med. Fat Meat
Regular Roast Beef	5.2 oz	353	32	22	15	590	2 Starch/Bread, 2 Med. Fat Meat, 1 Fat
Hot Ham 'n Cheese Sandwich	5.7 oz	353	33	26	13	1655	2 Starch/Bread, 3 Med. Fat Meat
Turkey Deluxe	7 oz	375	32	24	17	850	2 Starch/Bread, 3 Med. Fat Meat
Roasted Chicken Boneless Breast	5 oz	254	2	43	7	930	6 Lean Meat
Roasted Chicken Boneless Leg	5.35 oz	319	1	41	16	995	6 Lean Meat
Tossed Salad w/Low-Calorie Italian Dressing	8 oz	57	8	3	1	465	1 Vegetable
Baked Potato, Plain	11 oz	290	66	8	1	12	4 Starch/Bread
BURGER KING							
Hamburger	1	275	29	15	12	509	2 Starch/Bread, 2 Med. Fat Meat
Cheeseburger	1	317	30	17	15	651	2 Starch/Bread, 2 Med. Fat Meat, 1 Fat
Chicken Tenders	6 pieces	204	10	20	10	636	1 Starch/Bread, 2 Med. Fat Meat
French Fries	Regular	227	24	3	13	160	1½ Starch/Bread, 2 Fat
Salad w/Reduced Italian Dressing	1	42	7	2	trace	449	1 Vegetable
BK Broiler	1	379	31	24	18	764	2 Starch, 3 Med. Fat Meat
DAIRY QUEEN							
Single Hamburger	1	360	33	21	16	630	2 Starch/Bread, 2 Med. Fat Meat, 1 Fat
Single w/cheese	1	410	33	24	20	790	2 Starch/Bread, 3 Med. Fat Meat, 1 Fat

(Cont.)

164

(*Cont.*)

Product	Serving size	Calories	Carbo-hydrates (grams)	Protein (grams)	Fat (grams)	Sodium (milli-grams)	Exchanges
DAIRY QUEEN (*Cont.*)							
Fish Fillet	1	430	45	20	18	674	3 Starch/Bread, 2 Med. Fat Meat, 1 Fat
French Fries	Regular	200	25	2	10	115	1½ Starch/Bread, 2 Fat
Frozen Dessert*	4 oz	180	27	4	6	65	2 Starch/Bread, 1 Fat
Cone*	Regular	240	38	6	7	80	2½ Starch/Bread, 1 Fat
Dilly Bar*	1	210	21	3	13	50	1½ Starch/Bread, 2 Fat
*For occasional use only							
DOMINO'S PIZZA							
Cheese Pizza 12-inch	2 slices	340	52	18	6	660	3 Starch/Bread, 1 Med. Fat Meat, 1 Vegetable
Pepperoni Pizza 12-inch	2 slices	380	48	20	12	880	3 Starch/Bread, 2 Med. Fat Meat, 1 Vegetable
HARDEE'S							
Hamburger	1 (96 gm)	276	21	14	15	589	1½ Starch/Bread, 1½ Med. Fat. Meat, 1 Fat
Grilled Chicken Sandwich	1	310	34	24	9	890	2 Starch, 3 Lean Meat
Roast Beef Sandwich	1 (129 gm)	312	30	20	12	826	2 Starch/Bread, 2 Med. Fat Meat
Chef Salad	1 (336 gm)	227	10	23	16	517	2 Vegetable, 3 Med. Fat Meat
KENTUCKY FRIED CHICKEN							
Original Recipe Wing	1 (56 gm)	181	6	12	12	387	½ Starch/Bread, 1½ Med. Fat Meat, 1 Fat
Side Breast	1 (96 gm)	276	10	20	17	654	½ Starch/Bread, 3 Med. Fat Meat
Center Breast	1 (107 gm)	257	8	26	14	532	½ Starch/Bread, 3 Med. Fat Meat
Drumstick	1 (58 gm)	147	4	14	9	269	2 Med. Fat Meat
Thigh	1 (96 gm)	278	8	18	19	517	½ Starch/Bread, 2 Med. Fat Meat, 2 Fat
Kentucky Nuggets	6 (96 gm)	276	13	17	17	840	1 Starch/Bread, 2 Med. Fat Meat, 1 Fat

(*Cont.*)

Product	Serving size	Calories	Carbo-hydrates (grams)	Protein (grams)	Fat (grams)	Sodium (milli-grams)	Exchanges
KENTUCKY FRIED CHICKEN (*Cont.*)							
Hot Wings	6	376	18	22	24	677	1 Starch/Bread, 3 Med. Fat Meat, 2 Fat
Mashed Potatoes w/Gravy	1 (86 gm)	62	10	2	1	297	1 Starch/Bread
Corn-on-the-Cob	1 (143 gm)	176	32	5	3	21	2 Starch/Bread
Cole Slaw	1 (79 gm)	103	12	1	6	171	2 Vegetable or 1 Starch/Bread, 1 Fat
Baked Beans	1 (89 gm)	105	18	5	1	387	1 Starch/Bread
LONG JOHN SILVER'S							
Baked Fish Dinner w/slaw, mixed veg.	1	387	19	36	19	1298	1 Starch/Bread, 4 Med. Fat Meat
Shrimp Salad w/crackers	1	183	12	27	3	658	1 Starch/Bread, 3 Lean Meat
Ocean Chef Salad w/crackers	1	222	9	28	8	983	1 Starch/Bread, 3 Lean Meat
A La Carte: Kitchen-Breaded Fish	1 (2 oz)	122	8	9	6	374	1 Starch/Bread, 1 Med. Fat Meat
Catfish Fillet	1 (2.7 oz)	203	13	12	12	469	1 Starch/Bread, 1 Med. Fat Meat, 1 Fat
Tender Chicken Plank	1 (2.2 oz)	152	10	9	8	515	1 Starch/Bread, 1 Med. Fat Meat
Battered Scallops	3 pc. (2.1 oz)	159	12	6	9	603	1 Starch/Bread, 1 High Fat Meat
Breaded Oysters	3 pc. (2.1 oz)	180	18	6	9	195	1 Starch/Bread, 1 High Fat Meat
Battered Shrimp	3 pc. (1.8 oz)	141	9	6	9	462	1 Starch/Bread, 1 High Fat Meat
Clam Chowder	6.6 oz	128	15	7	5	611	1 Starch/Bread, 1 Med. Fat Meat
Hushpuppies	2 pc. (1.7 oz)	145	18	3	7	405	1 Starch/Bread, 1½ Fat

(*Cont.*)

166

(Cont.)

Product	Serving size	Calories	Carbo-hydrates (grams)	Protein (grams)	Fat (grams)	Sodium (milli-grams)	Exchanges
McDONALD'S							
Hamburger	1 (100 gm)	263	28	12	11	506	2 Starch/Bread, 1 Med. Fat Meat, 1 Fat
Quarter Pounder	1 (160 gm)	427	29	25	23	718	2 Starch/Bread, 3 Med. Fat Meat, 1 Fat
Chicken McNuggets	6	288	17	19	16	520	1 Starch/Bread, 2 Med. Fat Meat, 1 Fat
French Fries, small	1 (68 gm)	220	26	3	12	109	2 Starch/Bread, 2 Fat
Egg McMuffin	1 (138 gm)	340	31	19	16	885	2 Starch/Bread, 2 Med. Fat Meat, 1 Fat
Scrambled Eggs	1 (98 gm)	180	2	13	13	205	2 Med. Fat Meat, 1 Fat
English Muffin w/butter	1 (63 gm)	186	30	5	5	310	2 Starch/Bread, 1 Fat
Apple Bran Muffin	1	190	46	5	0	230	3 Starch/Bread
PIZZA HUT							
Thin-n-Crispy cheese 10-inch	1/2	450	54	25	15	*	3½ Starch/Bread, 2 Med. Fat Meat, 1 Fat
Thin-n-Crispy Supreme 10-inch	1/2	510	51	27	21	*	3 Starch/Bread, 3 Med. Fat Meat, 1 Fat
Thick-n-Chewy Pepperoni 10-inch	1/2	560	68	31	18	*	4½ Starch/Bread, 3 Med. Fat Meat

*Not available.

Product	Serving size	Calories	Carbo-hydrates (grams)	Protein (grams)	Fat (grams)	Sodium (milli-grams)	Exchanges
RAX							
Roast Beef Sandwich	Regular	320	33	20	11	969	2 Starch/Bread, 2 Med. Fat Meat, 1 Fat
Ham & Swiss Sandwich	1 (224 gm)	430	42	23	23	1737	3 Starch/Bread, 2 Med. Fat Meat, 2 Fat
Plain Potato	1 (250 gm)	270	60	8	trace	70	4 Starch/Bread
French Fries, small	1 (3 oz)	260	33	2	13	69	2 Starch/Bread, 2 Fat
Cream of Broccoli Soup	3.5 oz	50	6	1	2	219	½ Starch/Bread
Chicken Noodle Soup	3.5 oz	40	8	2	trace	40	½ Starch/Bread

(Cont.)

167

Product	Serving size	Calories	Carbo-hydrates (grams)	Protein (grams)	Fat (grams)	Sodium (milli-grams)	Exchanges
(Cont.)							
SHAKEY'S							
Thin Cheese 13-inch pizza	1/10	140	18	9	5	315	1 Starch/Bread, 1 Med. Fat Meat
Thin Onion, Green Pepper, Olive, Mushroom 13-inch pizza	1/10	171	21	10	5	395	1 Starch/Bread, 1 Med. Fat Meat, 1 Vegetable
Thick Pepperoni 13-inch pizza	1/10	232	19	19	8	494	1 Starch/Bread, 2 Med. Fat Meat
TACO BELL							
Bean Burrito	1	343	48	11	12	272	3 Starch/Bread, 2 Fat
Beef Burrito	1	466	37	30	21	327	2½ Starch/Bread, 3 Med. Fat Meat, 1 Fat
Beef Tostada	1	291	21	19	15	138	1½ Starch/Bread, 2 Med. Fat Meat, 1 Fat
Bellbeefer	1	221	23	15	7	231	1½ Starch/Bread, 1½ Med. Fat Meat
Taco	1	186	14	15	8	79	1 Starch/Bread, 2 Lean Fat Meat
WENDY'S							
Single Hamburger patty on white bun	1 (127 gm)	350	26	24	16	360	2/Bread, 3 Med. Fat Meat
Plain Baked Potato	1 (250 gm)	250	52	6	2	60	3½ Starch/Bread
Chili	9 oz (256 gm)	230	16	21	9	960	1 Starch/Bread, 3 Lean Meat
Fish Fillet	1 (92 gm)	210	13	14	11	475	1 Starch/Bread, 2 Med. Fat Meat
Taco Salad	1 (791 gm)	660	46	41	37	1110	3 Starch/Bread, 5 Med. Fat Meat, 1 Fat
Pick Up Window Salad	1 (579 gm)	110	5	8	6	540	1 Vegetable, 1 Fat
Garden Spot Salad Bar: Lettuce, Iceberg	3 cups	20	3	trace	trace	20	1 Vegetable

(Cont.)

(Cont.)

Product	Serving size	Calories	Carbo-hydrates (grams)	Protein (grams)	Fat (grams)	Sodium (milli-grams)	Exchanges
WENDY'S (*Cont.*)							
Pasta Salad	¼ cup	130	18	3	6	190	1 Starch/Bread, 1 Fat
Sunflower Seeds & Raisins	1 oz	140	6	5	10	5	½ Fruit, 1 High Fat Meat
Reduced-Calorie Italian Dressing	2 Tbsp.	45–50	2	trace	4–5	140–180	1 Fat
ZANTIGO							
Taco	1 (84.5 gm)	198	13	10	12	318	1 Starch/Bread, 1 Med. Fat Meat, 1 Fat
Taco Burrito	1 (198.7 gm)	415	41	21	19	815	2½ Starch/Bread, 2 Med. Fat Meat, 2 Fat
Hot Cheese Chilito	1 (115.3 gm)	329	35	14	15	466	Starch/Bread, 1 Med. Fat Meat, 2 Fat

This chart is excerpted from a more extensive version in Fast Food Facts. *See Resources.*

169

- Pizza is a good fast food choice, and it provides valuable nutrients to your diet as well. The best choice is cheese pizza with vegetables. Other toppings, such as pepperoni, sausage, and extra cheese, add calories, fat, and sodium. One word of caution: the high carbohydrate content of pizza can raise blood glucose levels excessively in some people. Self-monitoring your blood glucose levels periodically for 1 to 2 hours after eating pizza will help you learn whether it is a good fast food for you.

- When ordering hamburgers, stay away from the double burgers with cheese or sauces. Also, cheeseburgers have 100 more calories than hamburgers as well as extra fat and sodium.

- Stay away from "super" hot dogs with cheese or chili. These are very high in calories and sodium.

- Choose chicken or fish only if it is roasted, unbreaded, grilled, baked, or broiled without fat. Chicken or fish that is battered, breaded, or fried is higher in calories and fat than a hamburger. Also, stay away from mayonnaise-based sauces.

- Try to order regular or junior size sandwiches rather than the larger, top-of-the-line deluxe types. You san save calories by skipping the mayonnaise and adding lettuce, tomato, onion, and mustard instead.

- Choose plain lean roast beef, turkey or chicken breast, or lean ham. To save additional fat and calories, choose a bun or bread instead of a croissant.

- Choose a salad, but be careful with high-fat toppings like dressings, bacon bits, cheeses, and seeds. Load up on lettuce and vegetables at a salad bar, and go easy on the dressing, croutons, mayonnaise, and macaroni salads. Even too much low-calorie salad dressing can make a difference. So, check the number of calories on the packet.

- Order tacos, tostados, bean burritos, soft tacos, and other nonfried items when eating in Mexican fast food restaurants. Choose chicken items over beef and avoid beans if they are refried in lard (ask whether they are made with lard). Pile on extra lettuce, tomatoes, and salsa. Go easy on cheese toppings and fillings, sour cream, and guacamole. Limit your intake of the deep-fried taco salad shell—a taco salad can have more than 1,000 calories!

- Satisfy your sweet tooth with sugar-free nonfat frozen yogurt (only 80 calories in 1/3 cup) or a small ice milk cone. Ices, sorbets, and sherbets generally have less fat and fewer calories than ice cream but are a significant source of sugar and can raise your blood glucose level rapidly. Better still, bring a piece of fresh fruit from home!

- A healthy breakfast is the hardest meal to find in a fast food restaurant. Try a plain bagel, toast, or English muffin; be aware that other kinds of muffins can be loaded with sugar. Request no butter or margarine and low-sugar jam or jelly. Add fruit juice or low-fat or skim milk. Order cold cereals with skim milk, pancakes without butter, or plain scrambled eggs. If necessary, bring your own low-sugar jam and sugar-free syrup. Avoid bacon and sausage.

GROCERY SHOPPING AND READING LABELS

These days, with so many new products on the market, it's important to be an informed shopper. It's especially important for people with diabetes to know the ingredients of the products they buy.

Not all foods have nutrition labeling. Legally, it's required only when a product makes a nutritional claim like "high in protein," "low in sugar," or "fortified with vitamins." But with today's diet-conscious public, many products carry nutrition labels voluntarily. So, when you shop, read the nutrition panel that appears somewhere on the container.

The nutrition label lists the serving size, stated in common measurements for that product, such as ounces, cups, teaspoons, or even pieces. The label gives the number of servings per container. It also tells the calories per serving and the weight (in grams) of protein, carbohydrate, and fat per serving. It must list the percentage of the United States Recommended Daily Allowances (RDA) of vitamins A and C and certain other nutrients contained in that serving. Thus, if the label says there is thiamine 2, one serving of the product contains 2 percent of the RDA for thiamine.

If the package makes a claim about fat, such as "low cholesterol," it must identify the kind of fats it contains. Finally, the label usually shows milligrams of sodium (salt contains sodium, and sodium is also found in other compounds in food), and sometimes the milligrams of potassium in a serving.

Serving Size

It is important to note that the serving size is determined by the manufacturer. The law only requires that it be reasonable. A juice manufacturer cannot call 3 ounces a serving, because few would consider 3 ounces a reasonable serving of juice. Juice usually comes in 6-ounce servings.

Keep track of the number of servings in the container as you eat the product. You may have to adjust the calorie value and the grams of carbohydrate, protein, and fat if your portions are larger than the manufacturer's.

Exchanges

Your dietitian can teach you how to use the information on the nutrition label to calculate the exchanges for the amount of that food you want to eat. For instance, a product with 7 grams of carbohydrate, 2 grams of protein, and 5 grams of fat per serving is equal to about 1/2 Starch/Bread and 1 Fat exchange.

Additional Label Information

Sometimes the nutrition panel provides specific information about how many grams of carbohydrate are complex sugars and how many are simple sugars. That's valuable information for people with diabetes, who want to eat foods with complex, not simple sugars.

When you shop, remember that a nutrition label does not automatically make a product healthy. A highly sugared snack cake may carry a nutrition label because it claims to be enriched with added vitamins and minerals. Of course, nutrition labels are found only on prepackaged foods, and many foods without them are wholesome indeed. You'll never see a nutrition label on an orange.

Itemized Ingredients

Ingredient labels must appear on nearly every packaged food product. Reading the labels will enable you to know the relative amounts of each ingredient in the product and the kinds of specific sugars that may have been added.

Ingredients are listed according to their weight in the package, with the ingredient weighing the most listed first. For example, a food that puts sucrose as its first ingredient contains far more of this sugar than the same type of food that lists it seventh.

Decoding Food Labels

At the grocery store, you might be faced with deciding whether to buy the cereal shown in the sample label. When comparison shopping, be sure to check that serving sizes are equal. Also, be sure that the serving size is realistic. In the sample label, the serving size is one ounce, or approximately 2/3 cup. Is that how much cereal you eat?

Calorie count must be within 20 percent of actual calorie count. Thus, a serving of this product could contain anywhere from 88 to 132 calories.

All carbohydrates are lumped together. This listing includes simple sugars, complex carbohydrates, and fiber. Further explanation is optional (see below).

SAMPLE FOOD LABEL: ALL-NATURAL LOW-FAT CEREAL

Serving size	1 ounce
Calories	110
Protein	2 g
Carbohydrates	23 g
Total fat	6 g
Polyunsaturated fatty acid	4 g
Saturated fatty acid	2 g*
Cholesterol	0 mg
Sodium	180 mg
Potassium	55 mg

*Applies if coconut oil is used.

Percentage of U.S. Recomended Daily Allowance

Protein	4
Vitamin A	25
Vitamin C	*
Thiamine	25
Riboflavin	25
Niacin	25
Calcium	15
Iron	15
Vitamin D	10
Vitamin B_6	25
Folic Acid	25
Vitamin B_{12}	25
Phosphorus	4
Magnesium	4
Zinc	2
Copper	4

*Contains less than 2% of the U.S.R.D.A.

INGREDIENTS: Whole wheat, rolled oats, sugar, corn, brown sugar, partially hydrogenated soy bean and/or coconut oil, malted barley, salt, corn syrup, coconut, whey, malt syrup, honey, artificial flavor, artificial food coloring (Yellow No. 5), BHT, MSG.

Carbohydrate Information

Dietary Fiber	1 g
Complex carbohydrates	16 g
Sucrose and other sugars	6 g
Total carbohydrates	23 g

Ingredients are listed in descending order according to weight. But read carefully. Although this product contains whole wheat, rolled oats, and corn, it does not contain a lot of fiber. If you're anxious to increase fiber in your diet, this cereal would not be a wise choice.

The label does not have to specify which oil was actually used in this product. Low-fat products must list saturated and unsaturated fats as well as cholesterol.

If you add together the various forms of sweetener here (in this case, sugar, brown sugar, corn syrup, malt syrup, and honey), sweeteners become an important ingredient. Caloric sugars, like table sugar, provide four calories per gram, or approximately 120 calories per ounce of weight, regardless of their differences in sweetness. You can use some caloric sweeteners if they are approved by your dietitian or physician. Usually, the acceptable amounts of these sugars are those that will not cause a rapid rise in blood glucose to a high level. Products labeled "sugar free" may be very misleading. Many contain caloric sweeteners such as maltodextran or sorbitol that have as many calories as table sugar. Check the label for the amount of carbohydrate per serving and compare it to sugar-containing products.

Noncaloric sweeteners—aspartame (NutraSweet or Equal), acesulfame-K (Sweet One or Sunette), and saccharin (Sweet 'n Low, Sugar Twin, or Sweet 10)—are found in many products. It's best to discuss your use of noncaloric sweeteners and sugar-free products with your dietitian or physician.

Going Beyond the Label

Today, the lines have blurred between regular and "diet," "dietetic," "diabetic," or "health" items. Many sugar-free, low-calorie, low-fat, or low-sodium items sit alongside the regular products on supermarket shelves or in freezers. They usually cost about the same as their regular counterparts. A similar item in the special "diet" section of the store, however, usually costs more. Other products, such as egg substitutes, special ketchups, and low-sodium, sugar-free cookies, which also may be in a special section, are going to cost one-fourth to twice as much as their "regular" counterparts.

No matter where a food is placed on the supermarket shelf or what its price, it pays to read the ingredients list. Front labels on packages can be misleading. Products today are often marked "sugar free," "reduced calorie," "low sodium," or "natural" on the front of the package as a marketing strategy and not because they are truly better for you.

The words "dietetic" or "diet" on a product do not give enough information for you to make an informed choice. Remember that "dietetic" does not necessarily mean it's low in sugar. The word "dietetic" on a food label only means that something has been changed or replaced in that product. The item may contain less sugar, less sodium, less fat, or less cholesterol than the same "regular" product. If you look closely at the ingredients list of a package of dietetic cookies, you might find that they are only low in sodium and not low calorie or sugar free, as the name may imply.

Food and Drug Administration (FDA) regulations require that foods marked "low calorie" have no more than 40 calories per serving. "Reduced-calorie" items must contain at least one-third fewer calories than the regular product. Many words on the front label, however, are not limited by federal regulations. Currently, the FDA allows virtually any word to be used in the name or trademark of a product, even it it's misleading. For instance, if you think that "light" or "lite" always means fewer calories, that "natural" always means that nothing has been added, or that "low cholesterol" means the food is good for your heart, you are in for a surprise.

The words "no cholesterol" and "lite" are often misused. Liquid cholesterol-free vegetable oils are not fat free or calorie free. However, they do not have the saturated fat found in fats from animal sources; instead, they contain unsaturated fats. The word "lite" has been used indiscriminately. Food companies hope you'll pick the "lite" label, maybe even pay more for it, although the word is no guarantee that the product is going to be healthier than the regular version.

The word "natural" also has no clear definition except on meat and poultry products, where it means that no chemical preservatives, fillers, hormones, or the like have been added. On labels of other foods, the word "natural" is not restricted in its meaning by government regulatory requirements.

However, a food labeling revolution is in progress. The FDA has proposed new labeling regulations that standardize serving sizes, nutrient content claims (such as "low sodium"; "sugar free"; and "reduced," "less," or "light"), and health claims that address a specific disease. For instance, a food that calls itself "light" or "lite" must have one-third less calories and 50 percent less fat than an unmodified "normal" version. The proposal even includes making the labels state how much of the daily recommended intake of fat, carbohydrate, fiber, and sodium is contained in one serving, based on a 2,350-calorie daily diet.

An item advertised as low calorie because it contains artificial sweeteners may indeed be low calorie. Artificial sweeteners such as aspartame, acesulfame-K, and saccharin are much lower in calories than sucrose, which is regular table sugar. Products sweetened with these artificial sweeteners may help in weight loss. One example is Sugar-Free Jello Gelatin. A 1/2-cup serving may be used as a free item if you are on a low-calorie or low-fat meal plan. But, in general, it's best to check to see what ingredients the low-calorie product contains in addition to the low-calorie sweetener.

What about fiber? Every day we hear of new products with fiber, particularly oat bran. Again, read the ingredients list. How much oat or corn bran is actually in there? How much fat and sugar? And what other ingredients does the food contain? Most commercially made muffins and muffin mixes are loaded with fat and sugar. Cooking plain oat bran is the least expensive way to get the most fiber while taking in the smallest amounts of calories, sugar, fat, and sodium. If you prefer a ready-to-eat oat bran cereal, check the ingredients list for one with the highest amount of oat bran and smallest amounts of sugar and fat.

Shopping Smart

You'll probably discover your healthiest and most economical food choices by reading the ingredients list, not by reaching automatically for the specially marked items. Sometimes, however, certain specialty products may be worth the extra expense. They may save you time and reduce the stress of always doing without something you like.

Being an informed shopper will help you buy healthy food at reasonable prices.

It's best to shop the perimeter of the market first: usually grocery stores are organized so that the basic four food groups make up the four enclosing walls—produce, dairy, meat, and breads. Fill your cart with these nutritious essentials first, then proceed down only the aisles necessary to complete your grocery list.

- **Milk.** Look for skim or 1 percent milk. Buttermilk usually is made from skim milk, but check the label.

- **Yogurt.** Choose plain nonfat yogurt or fruited nonfat or low-fat yogurt sweetened with an artificial sweetener. Artificially sweetened yogurts are often labeled "lite" and are 50 to 100 calories per serving, depending on serving size.

- **Cheese.** Choose skim milk cheeses with about 5 grams of fat per ounce or less. Examples include Alpine Lace cheeses, Kraft Light Naturals cheeses, skim-milk mozzarella and farmer's cheeses, and most American-flavor cheeses, excluding pasteurized processed style. Nonfat ricotta cheese is also a good choice.

- **Bread.** Choose a bread that lists whole grains as the first ingredient on the label. Remember, two slices of diet (40-calories-per-slice) bread equal one Starch/Bread exchange.

- **Cereal.** Choose cereals listing "whole" grains as the first ingredient on the label. Look for cereals that have 2 or more grams of fiber and 1 gram or less of fat per serving. They should also provide less than 5 grams of sucrose or other sugars per serving.

- **Crackers.** Choose crackers made with whole grains or mostly whole grains. The best crackers have less than 2 grams of fat per serving, which is usually 5 to 12 (or 1 ounce of) crackers, depending on their size.

- **Rice, pasta, and whole grains.** Buy brown or wild rice of any type. Choose unfilled fresh or dried pasta, preferably made with whole wheat or vegetables, such as spinach, tomato, or artichoke. Most whole grains, such as bulgur wheat, wheat berries, or oat groats, contain 100 calories per 1/2 cup of cooked grain and no fat.

- **Red meat.** Beef, veal, and pork are usually labeled with animal name and body part and then type of cut; for instance, pork loin chops. Meat is graded Prime (highest in fat), Choice, or Select (lowest in fat). Choose select grades and lean body parts, such as the loin, tenderloin, round, or

177

leg. Also, ask your butcher to preportion the serving to 4 ounces of raw meat each.

- **Luncheon meat.** Choose lean or greater than 90 percent fat-free meats. They should contain 30 to 35 calories and about 1 gram of fat per ounce.

- **Poultry.** The leanest cut is boneless, skinless breast meat. Removing the skin cuts the fat in half and the cholesterol by 75 percent. Turkey or chicken processed as traditional pork-based meats, such as salami, bologna, hot dogs, and bacon, are still high in fat and should only be used occasionally. Use ground turkey breast the next time you cook hamburgers.

- **Fish.** Choose fresh fish or shellfish in the delicatessen case. The best choice in canned seafood is fish packed in water with no added salt. Select fresh or frozen fish without batter or breading.

- **Frozen entrees.** Look for dinner entrees that are 350 calories or less per serving. Ideally, fat should make up less than 30 percent of calories; this means the entrees would provide about 3 grams of fat per 100 calories—about 10 grams of fat per serving. Choose entrees with less than 800 milligrams of sodium and less than 100 milligrams of cholesterol per serving.

- **Soup.** Low salt and low fat are the keys here. Look for frozen or canned soups with less than 500 milligrams of sodium per serving, usually 1 cup, and that contain less than 30 percent of their calories from fat (see "How to Figure Fat").

- **Frozen desserts.** Choose a dessert that contains no more than 3 grams of fat per 4-ounce serving. Frozen yogurt or "light" ice cream fits in this category. Look for frozen fruit juice bars that have less than 70 calories per bar (and do not contain cream or coconut). All frozen desserts will equal one serving of fruit.

- **Fruit and fruit juice.** Buy fresh fruit or freshly squeezed 100 percent fruit juice. As long as it's 100 percent (or pure) juice, it can be fresh or from concentrate, canned, bottled, or frozen. Beware of juice labels starting, "**made with** 100 percent juice"—this means the drink contains ingredients (probably sugars) in addition to 100 percent juice.

- **Jams and jellies.** Choose fruit spreads, all-fruit jams, or low-sugar spreads. If you eat less than 2 teaspoons per day, you will not have to count it in your calorie total.

- **Margarine and oil.** The first ingredient on the label should be a liquid vegetable oil. The oil should start with an "s" (soybean, safflower, sesame, or sunflower) or a "c" (corn or canola). Look for margarines and oils that contain no more than 1 gram of saturated fat per serving, usually a tablespoon. Be careful to monitor your portions of "light" and "diet" margarines or you could end up using two to three times what you normally would.

- **Salad dressings and sour cream.** Try to choose salad dressings that contain 30 calories or less per tablespoon. They are usually labeled as reduced-calorie salad dressings and can be used in 2-tablespoon servings versus the usual 1-tablespoon serving for regular salad dressings. Any oil-free salad dressing (usually 6 calories or less per tablespoon) may be used more liberally. Light sour cream substitutes still contain fat, and many are half sour cream. As long as amounts are monitored, sour cream as a fat exchange may be used (about 2 tablespoons equals a serving). If fat, cholesterol, and calories are of major concern, just use plain yogurt flavored with chives, herbs, and spices.

- **Cookies.** Choose cookies that contain about 60 to 80 calories per ounce (10 calories or less per cookie) and that have 2 grams or less of fat per ounce.

How to Figure Fat

Finding low-fat foods is one of the most important things you can do for your good health. Of all your daily calories, only about 30 percent should be from fat. Here are two ways to determine whether a product meets this guideline, using information given on the label.

Find the number of calories per serving and the grams of fat per serving. Then multiply the grams of fat by 9 and divide by the number of calories. When you multiply by 100, you'll have the percent of calories in that food supplied by fat. Here's a quick rule of thumb: a food that has less than 3 grams of fat

How to Figure Fat	
If calories per serving are between	Fat per serving should be *less* than
0 and 50	2 grams
50 and 100	3 grams
100 and 150	5 grams
150 and 200	7 grams
200 and 250	8 grams
250 and 300	10 grams
300 and 350	11 grams
350 and 400	13 grams
400 and 450	15 grams
450 and 500	17 grams

for every 100 calories is desirably low in fat. It's not unusual to find cookies and other desserts marketed to people with diabetes that have more than 60 percent of their calories from fat! A good choice at a vending machine would be a package of sourdough hard pretzels, which typically contains one serving of pretzels of 110 calories with less than 1 gram of fat.

Once you're familiar with these guidelines, you can feel safer choosing from the wide variety of convenience foods available at the grocery store. Just remember not to skip any of the food groups recommended in your daily meal plan.

Dealing With
Your Feelings

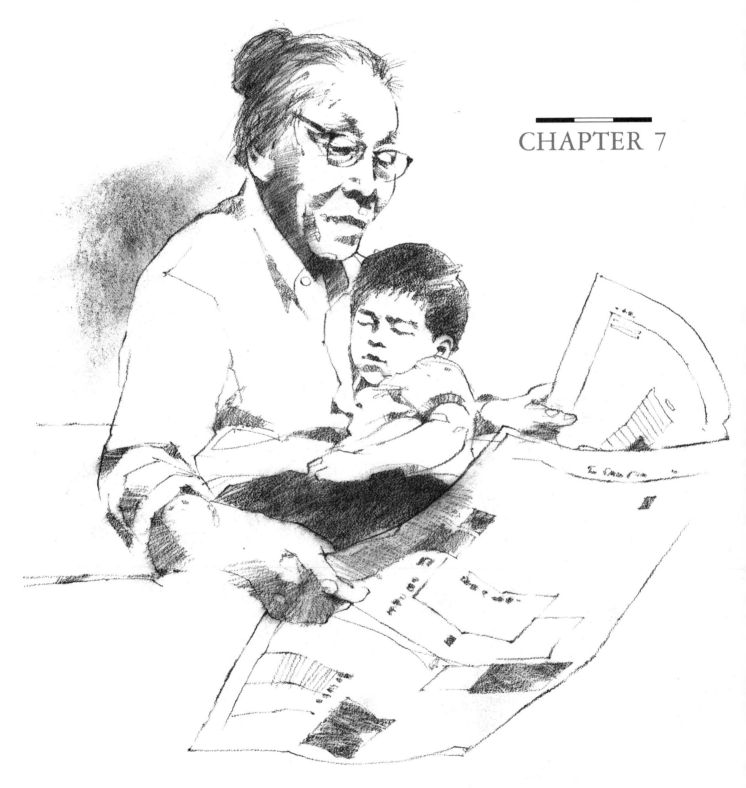

CHAPTER 7

Creating Your Support Network

There is strength in numbers. You don't have to face diabetes alone. Your family and your health-care team can help. So can your community. Most likely, it offers services that can help you manage your diabetes. Community service professionals can help you feel better about your health and about yourself. No matter where you live—city or country, farm or apartment—there are people and groups ready to help with your diabetes problems.

American Diabetes Association

One place to start is your local chapter or affiliate of the American Diabetes Association. There are 54 ADA Affiliates with a chapter or support group in 800 communities throughout the United States and Puerto Rico. Check the white pages of your phone book for the ADA presence nearest you.

Many chapters and affiliates will be happy to mail you a free packet of information on request. If you have questions about health insurance, Medicare, or Medicaid, you can get help finding the answers. If you have specific questions about diabetes, you can get books, brochures, and other information. And each month, *Diabetes Forecast* magazine has up-to-date medical, meal planning, and exercise information and tips for living with diabetes. A subscription to *Diabetes Forecast* is just one of the benefits of membership in the ADA. Cookbooks filled with healthy recipes and meal planning tips are also available. A list of ADA publications and other resources important to people with type II diabetes can be found near the end of this book.

If you've just learned that you have diabetes, ADA Affiliates and chapters can provide you with information you'll need to know. Many can refer you to doctors, diabetes educators, dietitians, and other health-care professionals in your area. The people of the ADA understand your problems and will offer help and encouragement. The ADA can also direct you to a diabetes education program recognized for its quality.

Many ADA Affiliates and chapters sponsor support and educational groups you can join. These groups can help you deal with the emotional part of living with diabetes. Through such groups, you can meet other people with diabetes and talk with health-care experts. They can help you learn about nutrition, exercise, and medications.

What Your Family Can Do

To be successful at controlling your diabetes, you will need to enlist your family's cooperation. It's important for you to feel you are not alone in meeting the challenge of having diabetes.

First, each family member needs to understand what diabetes is, how it is controlled, and how to handle those rare emergencies. There are books, magazines, pamphlets, libraries, support groups, and medical professionals that can help. Family members should attend diabetes education classes, either with you or on their own. Ask them to go along to some of your doctor's appointments and to keep a running list of questions or topics they may wish to discuss with your primary care physician, dietitian, or diabetes educator.

Second, your family will probably need to change the foods it eats and when it eats. It's important for everyone to eat well-balanced meals at regular times. Although many people object to being on a special diet, in most cases the meal plan for people with diabetes is more "common sense" than "special." Large amounts of sugar, fats, and salt aren't good for anyone.

Third, along with good nutrition, exercise is important for diabetes control. Caring for your own health along with family members may be a way for all of you to get closer. You might exercise, bike, swim, or take long walks together. Soon, this new team effort just might add to the quality of life for all family members!

Your Partner May Need Support, Too

Partners may sometimes feel stressed out from the demands placed on them. If you shut them out of your diabetes care, they may feel a sense of helplessness in not being able to "rescue" you. If you shift an unreasonable amount of responsibility for your diabetes care onto them, they may resent that so much of their time and energy is spent to help you.

It can be frustrating and worrisome for your mate if you don't always make the effort to eat appropriately, monitor blood glucose levels, and exercise regularly. However, both of you need to realize that no one is perfect! It's also important for both of you to acknowledge that your feelings exist, whatever they are, and to share them honestly. Communicating, rather

183

than denying or suppressing, your feelings may help bring you closer.

Sharing feelings with others is often crucial. Admitting that either or both of you may need help is a sign of strength, not weakness. Confide in your friends. Speak with your spiritual counselor. Consider speaking with professional counselors who are trained in chronic disease coping skills. Your health-care team members or your state ADA Affiliate will give you the names of people to call.

Finally, don't forget humor. Laughter helps lighten our load; it relaxes us.

Suggestions for Family Members

Caring about someone who has diabetes offers special challenges in addition to the usual ones.

- Get an education in diabetes care.

- Be supportive, but not a caretaker.

- Help someone you love keep to the rules, not break them.

- Lend a sympathetic ear.

- Stay flexible; be open to new ways of eating and spending free time.

- Plan for emergencies.

WORKING IT OUT

Our 30-year marriage has been a solid one, probably better than most. We brought up three children and weathered teenage rebellion and financial setbacks. Amazingly, it's diabetes that has nearly torn apart the fabric or our marriage. Joe insisted on denying his illness; I gradually became a shrill, anxious nag.

We decided to take a week's vacation to get our marriage back on track. Joe, who was put on insulin after trying to control his diabetes with diet and exercise, had four bad low blood glucose reactions during the trip. The worst happened as we were ambling happily around an interesting little town. In a panic, I realized that we didn't have any food with us.

(Cont.)

(Cont.)

I grabbed his arm and dragged him to the nearest restaurant. I was sure that people thought he was either drunk or stoned. I looked around and saw only indifference and hostility.

"My husband is diabetic," I said. "Please bring a hamburger and soda right away." But I felt, probably irrationally, that they didn't believe me, didn't care, and probably wouldn't help me. He downed a soda and was soon all right.

"Why are you so angry?" he asked.

"I'm not angry," I replied, "just sad, so sad." We were pretty quiet the rest of the trip.

The night we got home, we were each immersed in a book. Suddenly, Joe, who has great difficulty talking about emotions, looked at me and said, "Let's talk. I think you hate me."

I burst into tears and everything poured out. Joe thought that I was always angry at him, that I hated his illness and hated him. He always supported me when I was ill; why couldn't I do the same for him? What about our vows about sustaining each other in sickness and in health? And I told Joe how frustrated, anxious, and unappreciated I felt.

We talked and wept and talked some more. And suddenly all the anger and the hurt and the misunderstanding began to dissipate.

I don't pretend that we're out of the woods yet, but everything is so much better. Joe's finally accepted his denial and how dangerous and harmful it is. He seems finally to understand my anxiety and has begun to look on me as a concerned companion instead of a nag.

For my part, I've tried to understand how he chafes at being dependent on me and how it hurts him when I am angry and hostile. And I've stopped worrying so much about what people think. Above all, we've learned how essential it is to talk to each other when problems come up.

—*Joanna Martin, Los Angeles, California*

- Make sure others know how to recognize and care for hypoglycemia.

- Keep an optimistic, positive attitude.

- Remember that humor can help all of you through tough situations.

- Know that your feelings are valid and that they count.

- Don't strive for perfection in yourself or others; work for balance in your life.

Psychotherapy

Sometimes, sharing your feelings with those close to you isn't enough or doesn't seem to lead to solutions. You might be able to move ahead in working out your difficulties if you seek a professional, objective source of support. Professional psychotherapy will help you examine your problems. Depending on the nature of your needs, you may want individual, marriage, or family therapy.

Psychotherapy involves an ongoing conversation between you and the therapist. You will explore your thoughts and feelings and examine your interactions with others and the decisions you make. Starting at the "beginning" in telling your story to someone new may help you find a new viewpoint on the problems in your life and discover the patterns in your actions. The therapist will offer suggestions for considering situations from another person's perspective or trying new ways of coping. This may include learning to change negative thinking about yourself and correcting poor habits through self-awareness and rewards.

It is important to find a therapist with whom you feel comfortable and who is supportive. You may need to talk to several before it feels right. See Resources for professional organizations that can make local referrals.

Psychotherapy of any kind is an opportunity to become better acquainted with yourself. Living with diabetes means adjusting to the complex interplay between family relations, personality, emotions, and blood glucose control. The key to psychotherapy is to desire to make changes in your behavior. Therapy will help you to keep from being "stuck" in your old, perhaps destructive, behavior patterns.

Consider Group Therapy

Weekly group therapy sessions foster mutual support and help combat depression and isolation. A well-run therapy group provides a safe and accepting environment in which to talk about life with diabetes. Sometimes it's easier to find solutions to our problems when we share them with other people.

Groups meet in all types of settings, from hospitals and clinics to community agencies and therapists' private offices. Group therapy includes a trained therapist, a careful selection of group members, and a social structure that includes rules for behavior. All psychotherapy groups share the principle that talking about feelings, ideas, and experiences in a safe, respectful atmosphere increases self-esteem, deepens self-understanding, and helps a person get along better with others.

The group setting gives each member a chance to see how others react to their feelings about diabetes and observe how they incorporate diabetes into family, work, and play. Group therapy has specific advantages for people with diabetes. It can help you

- Learn that you are not alone.

- Discuss deeper feelings, worries, and concerns that you may never have dreamed of mentioning elsewhere.

- Discover new approaches to old problems.

- Explore who you are and who you are not.

- Reduce stress, which in turn may lead to more stable blood glucose levels, eating patterns, and exercise regimens.

187

EMOTIONS AND DIABETES

How do you feel about having diabetes? Do you feel angry and resentful? Do the added burdens of good self-care and extra medical bills make your already too stressful life even harder? Do you feel differently now than you did when you were first told you have type II diabetes? Has diabetes made anything about your life better?

Although many people with diabetes may have similar feelings, each of us chooses different ways of responding to them.

Denying that diabetes is a serious disease is a choice some people make. Others choose to keep haphazard control of diabetes. Sometimes, people choose to fight stress in ways that actually worsen the problem. They may turn to alcohol, prescription medications, illegal drugs, caffeine, nicotine, or anything that will either give them a lift or calm them.

Some choose food binging as a way to fill the empty space inside. In fact, any excessive behavior, even gambling or oversleeping, may be a way to deal with stress.

Although few of these solutions work for anyone, because you have diabetes, most of them are dangerous from the word "go." They alter diabetes control and can dramatically endanger your health. Learning as much as possible about diabetes, becoming an expert in dealing with your body's responses to your feelings, and following the advice of your health-care team are much healthier choices.

Stress and Diabetes

Stress is a part of life for everyone. There are external pressures, such as deadlines, ringing telephones, traffic tie-ups, and family feuds. There are also internal pressures. Stress is our own internal response to the situation of the moment as well as to messages recorded within us a long time ago. Because much of stress comes from within, we can often control it. But it takes work.

The belief that there is a causal connection between psychological stress and poor diabetes control isn't new. People with diabetes, as well as doctors, have long suspected the relationship. Although there is no evidence that a stressful lifestyle can cause any disease, it is possible that stress can bring on symptoms in someone already headed for a disease. And in people diagnosed with diabetes, stress can affect blood glucose levels.

Stress affects diabetes control by way of "stress hormones." These hormones make stored energy like glucose and fatty acids available to the body in what's called the "fight or flight" response. When you do not have diabetes, that glucose can be used immediately. Insulin is able to let the glucose into the cells, where it can function as a fuel for the body.

When you have diabetes, however, insulin can't always let glucose into the cells, so the newly released glucose accumulates in the blood. Certain stress hormones (called catecholamines; an example is adrenalin) can actually decrease insulin release in type II diabetes, where some insulin secretion is normally still present. Obviously, learning to limit your stress might be helpful in controlling your blood glucose levels.

Although doctors have long known that stress management is a factor in long-term control of diabetes, new research shows that it can have significant rapid effect on blood glucose levels in type II diabetes. It is likely that new techniques as well as new drugs that help reduce stress will play an increasingly important role in future diabetes treatment.

Personality Types

In learning to handle stress, it's important to realize that not everyone finds the same things stressful and not everyone responds to stress the same way. You've probably heard about type A and type B behavior personalities. These personality types are one way to contrast people's varying responses to situations, to other people, and even to their own thoughts.

Type A folks are usually in a hurry. They're impatient with themselves and others and tend to overschedule and do more than one thing at a time. Type A's are often competitive and are likely to be perfectionists.

On the other hand, type B personalities rarely feel the urgency of time. They pace themselves, don't overreact, and can say "no" if they're too busy to take on a new assignment. They're usually modest about their achievements and don't need to produce to feel good about themselves.

Of course, most of us have some type A as well as type B characteristics. But these personality types make it easy to see that stress is created by the way we react to a situation, not by the situation itself.

Having diabetes can churn up real, imagined, or expected stresses in all of us. It can make you feel your body is no longer under your control. It may cause anger (why me?), guilt (I must have done something wrong), denial (I don't believe this is happening to me), depression (I feel sad and hopeless), or helplessness (I can't cope with this) or lower your self-esteem (something must be wrong with me). Such stressful thoughts can have a powerful effect on your body.

Diabetes can bring on stressful external situations, too. These might include the way friends, family, or coworkers perceive you and your disease; the cost of medical care; dietary limitations; the need to carry supplies everywhere; and the sight of people with diabetic complications. If you take insulin, you may find injections stressful. Your need to exercise and lose weight may be hard to deal with.

Although maintaining control over the disease is important for people with diabetes, setting impossible treatment goals or trying too hard isn't a good idea. It can lead to more stress. If you are a type A personality and expect to deal absolutely perfectly with diabetes, you're setting yourself up for a high-anxiety scenario.

Managing Stress

First, learn to recognize how you act when you're stressed out. Do you laugh nervously or are you frequently self-critical? Are you easily discouraged or find that you go through periods of frustration or boredom? Do you cry easily? Do you feel emptiness or apathy? Do you reject help from those close to you or demand unrealistic attention from them?

Then, try to discover what is causing your body to feel stressed. Diabetes testing can help you. Test your blood glucose levels when you are in—or have just come out of—a stressful situation. That will tell you how the event affected your blood glucose levels, which may help you understand what situations are stressful for you. (Not all stresses raise blood glucose levels, however.)

More insight might come from deciding whether you are more of a type A or type B personality. If you're type A, make a contract with yourself to slow down and to stop overcommitting your time. Get others to help out, and practice saying "no" when you feel like it. Allow extra hours to get things done and block out some time just for yourself.

Exercise is a natural ally against stress. Perhaps some of these stress-management tips will work for you.

- Find someone to talk to when something is bothering you.
- Join a support group.
- Form a discussion group on books, movies, or whatever interests you.
- Join a bowling league or get into a group sport.
- Start a potluck dinner group.

- Join a dance group—square dancing, jazz, folk, tap, ballroom.

- Take up a hobby like stamp or coin collecting or needlepoint.

- Exercise! Join a yoga or aerobics class.

- Learn to play a musical instrument.

- Volunteer to help others.

- Sign up for a class.

- Take minivacations, overnighters, or weekends away.

- Arrange for baby-sitters when you're home to allow for free time.

- Form a baby-sitting cooperative with other parents so you can get out more.

Everyone has choices in life. Pace yourself. Avoid excessive behavior. Make it a point to identify your stressors and do something about them. You may not be able to control traffic jams, an angry boss, or a crying baby, but you do have some control over your reactions to them. You even have control over how you react to your diabetes. Because you have diabetes, it

---

LEARNING TO RELAX

Progressive muscle relaxation therapy has helped people reduce stress and anger. It has also helped with stress-related conditions including headaches, anxiety, and some forms of high blood pressure.

The technique involves recognizing muscle tension by progressively tensing then relaxing various muscle groups. It is usually taught in a clinic by professionals. Sometimes, it is supplemented by a biofeedback procedure in which muscle tension, skin temperature, and other stress-sensitive body responses are electronically monitored. Usually the equipment gives off a sound that changes pitch or volume as the person relaxes or tenses. That sound tells the patient whether he or she is relaxing properly.

(Cont.)

(Cont.)

Although professional instruction is essential to achieve completely effective muscle relaxation, it's possible to adopt many of these relaxation techniques by yourself. Start with the facial muscles, then work down to your feet and toes. As you identify each group of muscles, tense them. Coordinate the tension with your breathing. Keep your eyes closed and imagine yourself relaxing.

- Close your eyes and breathe slowly and deeply.

- Inhale. Raise eyebrows. Tense them. Hold for the count of three. Relax eyebrows. Exhale.

- Inhale. Close mouth and eyes tightly. Squeeze. Hold for the count of three. Relax eyes and mouth. Exhale.

- Inhale. Bite down on teeth. Hold for count of three. Relax jaw. Exhale.

- Inhale. Pull shoulders up. Hold for count of three. Relax shoulders. Exhale.

- Inhale. Tense all muscles in the arms. Hold for count of three. Relax arms. Exhale.

- Inhale. Tense all muscles in the chest and abdomen. Hold for count of three. Relax muscles. Exhale.

- Inhale. Tense all muscles in the legs. Hold for count of three. Relax muscles. Exhale.

- Inhale. Tense all muscles in toes. Curl toes. Hold for count of three. Relax the muscles. Exhale.

- Keep your eyes closed for a short while. Gradually open them.

pays to look hard for healthy ways to deal with feelings of loneliness, low self-esteem, anger, other uncomfortable emotions, or outside pressures.

Building Self-Esteem

Self-esteem has a strong impact on every part of our lives. We do better in our work, studies, and personal relationships when

we have high self-esteem. And we are more likely to go after—
and obtain—what we want out of life when we have a strong
sense of ourselves and our own worth. Others are more likely to
think well of us also.

Much, although not all, of the way we feel and think about
ourselves comes from the way we interpret the messages,
spoken and unspoken, that parents and caregivers give us from
the time we are very young. From their treatment of us, we
begin to form an opinion of ourselves, an attitude about who
we are, and a sense of whether we like or dislike ourselves and
in what ways.

For instance, if you were not well coordinated as a child, you
might still feel that you are clumsy, unless your parent or
caregiver offsets that idea early, perhaps by appreciating other
qualities in you. However, the good news is that psychologists
feel that self-esteem is not fixed. In fact, within a certain
range, it fluctuates from day to day. We feel better or worse
about ourselves depending on things like

- How we think we look that day.

- How others respond to us.

- Our physical well-being.

- How prepared we are for the day's work.

- Whether we feel hopeful or hopeless about the future.

Where Does Diabetes Fit In?

It's harder to feel good about yourself when you have a chronic
disease like diabetes, but it's possible, and it's important to
try. On the physical side, blood glucose variations can affect
your mood, appetite, energy or fatigue level, sense of well-
being, and feeling of control over your life. Some people with
diabetes develop low self-esteem because they blame themselves
for having the illness. Or, they think less of themselves because
they feel different or wonder if there is something negative that
singled them out for this disease.

It's important to maintain a positive image of yourself.
Realize that everyone has to deal with some kinds of
limitations, both actual and believed. Don't be defeated by
what you think you don't have or can't do. Focus on your
pluses. Be generous with yourself, especially when no one else
is. The only thing stopping you from having a high self-esteem

is your own belief about yourself. Everyone has strengths, so emphasize yours.

When your self-esteem seems low, focus on things you like about yourself. You might like the way you dress, the handiwork you do, or your ability to appreciate and enjoy nature. You must refuse to be swallowed up by negative thoughts. One way to do this is by making a list of things that you like about yourself. If you can't compose such a list, get feedback from others. Keep the list handy for a day when your self-esteem is low. Participating in an activity you are usually successful or productive at or satisfied with can help. Then, tackle something you may be having difficulty with.

Negative Myths Can Work Against Us

Are you one of those people who cling to negative myths? Remember, although diabetes can't be cured, it can be controlled. To do this, it's important to discover any negative myths that may be getting in the way of your good diabetes control.

For instance, you may believe that you can't control your diabetes well because you lack the willpower necessary for good diabetes self-care. If you give into your desire for too much food or sweet snacks, you feed that image of yourself as undisciplined. Then you get upset with yourself, further lowering your self-esteem. Slowly, you begin to accept the fact that you have no willpower and are therefore unprepared and unable to take good care of your health.

However, everyone has the capacity to be disciplined and show restraint—you just need to find the proper motivation. Unfortunately, your negative view of yourself is likely to be a myth you have come to believe—a myth that is hurting your self-esteem. You can disprove such harmful myths in three steps.

- First, recognize them.

- Second, realize that they are myths rather than reality.

- Third, work—with help, if necessary—to change them.

Your self-esteem will probably increase when you discover new abilities you didn't know you have.

You Deserve to Be in Good Health

You can also raise your self-esteem by acting as if you deserve good health care. Taking your diabetes care regimen seriously will let others know it is important. When you monitor your blood glucose regularly, take your medication on time, do appropriate exercises, and stick with your meal plan—in short, if you act like you value yourself—your self-esteem is likely to go up. That, in turn, will make it more likely that you will continue to take good care of yourself.

Learning to Assert Yourself

Assertiveness is often confused with aggressiveness. Some people are afraid to say something assertively because they think that means they are domineering and pushy. Although it's true that both assertive and aggressive communications are direct and clear, they have different goals.

Aggressiveness aims to strip the listener of choices or alternatives. Although aggressive communication is direct, it is not always honest; it is always controlling.

Assertiveness, on the other hand, aims to open up choices and alternatives for both the speaker and the listener. Assertive communication is open and honest as well as direct.

Learning to assert yourself can lead to better communication and better diabetes control. Some people find it difficult to talk about their special diet or the time needed to care for their diabetes. Others are embarrassed to be different or to have their needs conflict with those of the people around them. Some simply find it difficult to call attention to themselves. Some people see social disapproval, job security, a doctor's impatience, or embarrassing attention as greater risks than admitting they need special attention. Speaking up is especially difficult in circumstances where it would be easier to keep quiet.

The risk that comes with discounting diabetes care in favor of social acceptability is too great to ignore. Because everyone's needs and perspectives are unique, any two people in a relationship—whether one of them has diabetes or not—will eventually run into some degree of conflict. This can occur between you and members of your health-care team, too. Your assertiveness—not aggressiveness—can help resolve such tensions and improve your care. If you don't understand or agree with a recommendation, say so and ask for explanations. Diabetes, which demands so much attention to be controlled, also presents an added challenge in a social situation or relationship as well as at the workplace.

You may wonder how much you have to disclose about your diabetes to make your needs known. The answer depends not only on the people but on the situations involved. Most situations can be smoothed over by good communications, including snacking and eating—or not eating—at appropriate times, no matter what companions are doing; monitoring blood glucose or giving an insulin injection at work or in a public place; admitting that you have hypoglycemia even when the situation makes it inconvenient; and getting quality medical care for diabetes.

Because of the pleasure and sociability of eating, it's particularly difficult to put health first at a social gathering involving food. But you must assert yourself and care for your diabetes needs. Try out these basic assertiveness skills.

■ **Learn to say "no."** A simple "no, thank you" communicates to yourself as well as to the person addressed that "I respect myself enough to act in my own best self-interest, and I respect you enough to know that you will understand."

■ **Maintain courtesy.** Courtesy is the premise on which assertive communication is built. It relays the assumption that you will treat your needs and those of others equally and that neither will suffer at the other's expense.

■ **Be direct.** Direct communication, while maintaining courtesy, is as important as saying "no" at the appropriate time.

■ **Watch others.** There are signals that other people project that will help you decide how to act with them. Some may be uncomfortable when you draw a blood sample for testing or inject insulin. But if the clock says it's time, respect yourself and find a way to do it.

■ **Stick with your timing.** Hypoglycemia is the most urgent situation in which you must be assertive. Don't put off treatment because you are in the middle of an interesting conversation or nearing the end of a long trail with a new hiking group.

- **Be firm.** It's important to be firm with yourself as well as with others. Decide that you need to forego particular foods, then, if pressed to join in, explain the fact simply and directly to others. Prepare your companions in advance about your diabetes care.

- **Maintain self-respect.** If you respect yourself, you will have no qualms about being assertive in explaining your situation ahead of time and asking for help should you need it.

Diabetes Can Challenge You to Increase Effective Communications

There is a right and wrong way to ask for help, whether from a companion on a hiking trip or from a doctor in his or her office. The way you ask can put you in a position of power or set you up as a victim. Feeling as though you actually have power in a given circumstance, rather than feeling you have to go along with other people's choices, will provide options and increase your control over your life.

For example, people often feel at the mercy of a doctor instead of realizing that it is a partnership. They discount the fact that they have an equal say in the direction their health care should take. As an assertive person, you can move from feeling trapped by other people and circumstances, such as diabetes, to a feeling of being in control.

HOSTAGE

On Saturday, January 24, 1987, I was teaching a makeup class in management accounting in the graduate program in business at Beirut University College. Within two hours of dismissing the class, three faculty colleagues and I were kidnapped by four men impersonating the Internal Security Forces of Lebanon.

My overriding problem during captivity was my diabetes. I had been diagnosed diabetic in 1967 and had been able to control my diabetes with pills and diet until 1982, when I was put on one NPH insulin injection a day.

(Cont.)

(Cont.)

The men who held us captive for so long had little or no understanding of diabetes mellitus. But to their credit, within 12 hours of taking us, the kidnappers asked us about the details of our medical needs. At the same time, my wife was arranging to have the information publicized in the local press and on television. It was not until Wednesday, however, that I was given insulin, syringes, and alcohol so that I could inject my daily requirements. During captivity, we changed locations and guards several times. Each of these changes called for a repetition of our explanations and prescriptions.

The problems of survival for a diabetic hostage were many: problems of communications, logistics, daily routine, meal schedules, lack of exercise, dietary needs, and unavailability of access to doctors as well as the usual diabetic concerns of hypo- and hyperglycemia, circulatory difficulties, infections, and worries about retinopathy. Fortunately, a few weeks back in the fresh air, with better diet and concerned professional medical attention, restored me to such a degree that I was able to withstand fairly radical surgical procedures for cancer of the larynx less than a month after my release.

I hope, by my example in surviving the rigors of more than three years as a hostage, to demonstrate that even those of us who have been treated as somewhat second-class citizens for so long can not only be survivors but can also be achievers even in the face of extreme adversity.

The good news is that in spite of our disease, in spite of its demands and limitations, in spite of our doctors' cautions, in spite of the frequent underestimates of our abilities, we are qualified, both mentally and physically, to contribute to society and its progress.

—*Robert B. Polhill, Arlington, Virginia*

Using assertive communication, you can make courteous, direct, and honest statements about your individual needs. You can create a feeling of confidence and equality in your interactions with others. You can keep your diabetes in good control without embarrassment or conflict.

To Have Good Diabetes Control, You Must Be Motivated

Some people think freedom means doing whatever, whenever they want. They decide to eat all the wrong foods in all the wrong amounts. Their blood glucose level remains high, they get sicker, and they are imprisoned by their diabetes.

But, at some point, they realize that only discipline can provide the tools to real freedom. Escaping from self-discipline actually prevents true freedom. By denying that they have diabetes, by running from the fact that they, at times, have a totally unhealthy lifestyle, and by trying to escape from taking care of their health, they ultimately sabotage their growth, pleasure, and life. What's free about that?

First, as you accept that you have diabetes, you will become free to apply the energy to deal with the disease, instead of wasting it on denial. Second, accept that you are responsible for your own choices. And, realize that you have a great many choices. Third, choose to maintain a healthy lifestyle because your diabetes has an effect on the other people in your life. Make it a positive one. Fourth, positive diabetes care demands that you delay your rewards for the appropriate time. You must delay certain pleasures—like eating something you want right now—because it helps you stay healthy. Fifth, you can have some flexibility if you balance diet, exercise, and medication in response to monitoring results.

You have many choices. You can regard diabetes as a challenge or a limitation. You can grow stronger and wiser or remain unhealthy. The choice you make makes all the difference.

199

ATTITUDE ADJUSTMENT

Okay. You say you're ready to manage your diabetes. Great! First, let's understand how your attitude toward having the disease helps you prioritize your diabetes care. It isn't always easy to make diabetes care a priority. Most of us juggle multiple responsibilities in our lives. Diabetes care can gradually fade to the back of our minds.

It may be helpful to first sit down and list all of your responsibilities. Then, prioritize them from most important to least important. You may want to reflect on what you will be able to accomplish in your life if you do not make your diabetes care your top priority.

Most of us struggle with maintaining diabetes self-care as our top priority. The use of our priority list can help us evaluate our own self-management approach. It may help us see how a change in priorities might lead to better diabetes control. Take some time to see if you can find any clues to your own attitude about how important diabetes self-care is for you.

Include the following considerations in your thinking. First, we all have freedom of choice. All choices have consequences. Following the diabetes self-care regimen closely is more likely to lead to good control, and it requires good organizational and assertiveness skills. Not following the diabetes self-care regimen does not require much effort, and it leads to poor health.

Second, we can create meaning out of our own lives. For instance, some people see having diabetes as a disaster. Others view it as a challenge. The good news is, because we put the meaning in the circumstances, we can also change that meaning when it is hurting us. Thus, diabetes care can be viewed as a challenge to be met by using good coping and organizational skills.

Third, we are born with a drive to learn and grow. Thus, if a strategy for improving adherence to our self-care regimen doesn't work the first time, we can reevaluate and try a new approach.

Recognizing Responsibility

Some people accept no responsibility for managing their own illness. They rarely accept the consequences of their actions, are uninterested in self-management, and seem overwhelmed by life. People expressing this behavior have little interest in caring for themselves, even in their personal hygiene and grooming. They generally feel helpless in the face of diabetes, so they don't act with a specific goal in mind.

These people have a "can't do it" attitude. They are extremely dependent on relatives and medical professionals to manage their disease for them. And because they feel they have no effect on anything, they'll say things like, "What's the use of following a diet? Nothing ever turns out right anyway." Or simply, "Diabetes has ruined my life."

If this behavior seems familiar to you, perhaps you feel defeated or overwhelmed. Talk things over with someone you trust. Decide whether you want to take an active role in your life. Decide whether you really want to give up. Creating a priority list is essential for you.

Other people act as though they can't make a difference in managing their diabetes. Unlike people who feel defeated, these people actively think of themselves as victims. They blame outsiders so much that they even feel happiness comes from the outside, rather than from something they earned or caused. They use the victim approach to manipulate the world. Their idea of making changes is by getting others to do what they want. Although they feel some personal responsibility, they don't look for solutions within themselves. Instead, they fight back by getting angry or by blaming others when things aren't going well.

For example, if they are having trouble with diabetes control, these people might blame their family, job, doctor, or medication instead of the way he or she handles diabetes. And, although a lot of complaining occurs, he or she makes no effort to change things at home or work or to communicate with the health-care team.

Are you are spending a great deal of energy finding others or outside causes to blame, feeling sorry for yourself, and not enjoying the moment? You should find someone to help you deal with your anger. It is obvious that you want to achieve good diabetes control, but you need to take on more personal responsibility. Try setting a small goal, such as keeping a food journal for one week. Have a back-up plan in case you fail, such as trying it again next week but just for three days. Ask someone to acknowledge your success or to help you cope if you miss your goal. Keep at it!

Other people find themselves saying, "I really eat too much and should lose 20 pounds, but my wife always cooks fried foods." Although they have a greater sense of fairness about the cause of their problems, they are still looking for someone else to share the blame.

These people are beginning to consider the difference between taking responsibility for their diabetes control and

201

leaving it to family and health-care professionals. However, too often they decide to avoid recognizing their own responsibilities. By finding real faults in others, however correct, they keep themselves from examining their own role. They tend to look closely at themselves only when things are going well.

Do you make lots of statements where you seem to accept responsibility, but then shift it to someone else? Do you find yourself saying, "I know I should talk to my doctor, but she's so difficult to reach"? Now is the time to reread your priority list. Decide just how much more effort you need to put forth to feel that you are doing your best to take care of your diabetes. Tell your doctor that you are having a hard time reaching her and work out solutions. Help your wife find recipes to prepare your favorite foods without frying. Take a good look at what you see as roadblocks and come up with constructive solutions. Then you'll know you're increasing your level of personal responsibility.

It may help to talk and think more about taking total responsibility for their your diabetes self-care. Look to yourself more than you do to others; try not to blame others for your unfortunate circumstances. You need not only to accept your responsibility but to act on your acceptance, too.

Once you have increased your responsibility to this level, you might hear yourself saying, "I need to lose weight, and I know it's up to me. I just haven't done it." Or, "I've been letting my control slip, and I need to improve."

Watch out for this hurdle; don't get stuck dwelling on the negative aspects of your diabetes, and don't spend time agonizing about complications that might occur in the future. Try to act on what's real, not what you fear. Put energy into changing what you can, and give up on what you can't change. You are close to maintaining good self-control of diabetes but are not quite there. Taking responsibility for your diabetes and listing good intentions are an excellent start. Realize that you must carry out those intentions to be effective. Here's how:

- Set a reasonable goal.

- Self-monitor your progress toward your goal.

- Ask for and receive feedback about your progress from health-care team members, family, and others close to you.

- Work to solve the problems that come up with constructive solutions; don't stop at just acknowledging the problems.

- Feel free to revise your goal to make it more appropriate for you.

- Build in a reinforcement system; contract with a friend or family member for a reward when your goal is reached.

Here are some signs that you're working toward taking total responsibility for your life: You understand your own contribution to your well-being and acknowledge your part when things don't go well. Because you have committed yourself to whatever effort is required to manage your diabetes, you are able to operate at your peak most of the time. You can act rather than waste resources or time in feeling sorry for yourself, blaming others, looking for excuses, or regretting mistakes.

Having total self-responsibility means that you seldom give in to social pressures to drink or overeat because others are doing it. If you make a mistake, use what you learn to act differently next time. What may be a crisis for someone who takes less personal responsibility is often an opportunity for growth.

When you keep the responsibility for diabetes care on yourself, you'll hear yourself saying things like, "Since developing diabetes, I have a new way of understanding how my body uses food." Or, "Diabetes has helped me realize how much I value feeling well." You know it's up to you to make things work out. If you get stuck,

- Monitor your progress; keep a journal; let your support group know how far along you are in achieving your goal.

- Look to yourself as your primary source of reinforcement, but ask for reinforcement from others as you need it.

- Work on tailoring your diabetes care regimen to your lifestyle; stay flexible.

The goal in diabetes self-management is to take responsibility for your own health care. Even if others have acted poorly or circumstances have not always worked out, it helps to know there is no profit in blaming others or looking outside yourself for solutions. Responsibility for diabetes self-management is not an easy goal to reach, no matter what your age or diabetes regimen.

Don't blame yourself for being at a low level of personal responsibility. This will just make you feel worse. Instead, realize that moving to a higher level of responsibility will come naturally when you begin to recognize your problems and are willing to try to solve them.

Don't Fall Into the Blood Glucose Level Trap

Some people fall into the trap of evaluating their diabetes self-management only on the basis of their blood glucose levels. Keep in mind that, although your behavior has much to do with your blood glucose levels, there are other factors that enter the picture. Things beyond your direct control—like differences from time to time in how steadily insulin enters your blood from the injection or how efficiently it works—can significantly affect your blood glucose level just as infections or unexpected stresses can.

Sometimes not even your doctor can find an explanation for high blood glucose levels. Accept that you can greatly influence your diabetes but you can't totally control the course it takes every minute. And don't blame yourself as soon as blood glucose level rises. Ask yourself some questions that might lead to an explanation. Consider what's in your power to change . . . and what's not.

Do You Ever Feel Guilty?

Guilt is an unpleasant feeling that can come from seemingly opposite causes. We feel guilty when we fail to do what we think we should do. Likewise, we feel guilty when we do the exact thing we know we should not do. If you have ever had an eating binge, stopped an exercise program right after you started it, or neglected your blood testing for a long time, you are probably well aware of how guilt can be related to diabetes self-care.

Not all guilt is harmful. Sometimes guilt can serve a useful purpose by prompting us to take corrective measures. Guilt can get us back on track and actually stimulate positive changes in our lives.

Guilt is harmful when it includes unhealthy levels of self-criticism and strong feelings of inadequacy. When this happens, self-confidence slips, and apathy about diabetes care can result. Excessive guilt can give us an attitude that evokes such thoughts as, "What's the use of trying? I know I am going to fail."

Keeping up with the multiple demands of diabetes care while meeting the other challenges of daily life is not easy. Some degree of failure, followed by guilt, is inevitable, regardless of how hard you try. The key is to learn to accept an occasional self-failure as an unavoidable part of having diabetes but still maintain the will to succeed.

Finding Support Can Help

When you feel guilty and at odds with yourself, remember that you do not have to face diabetes, or the emotions it brings, alone. Try asking family members or friends for support when the going gets tough. Commit yourself to joining or starting a support group.

People who live with diabetes have had to struggle. This struggle can help you develop sympathy toward other people's struggles, failures, and successes, which in turn can encourage a more forgiving attitude toward yourself. Forgiving yourself, evaluating why you fail at something, and taking and feeling pride in what you do well—even when you don't want to do it—all help to create a good self-image and a desire to take care of yourself. These can help you gain better diabetes control, and in the long run, they can make you feel better than constantly striving for perfection.

After all, you are human, just like everyone else!

It Helps to Have Reasonable Expectations

One way to avoid failure is to go slowly. It's unreasonable to make too many changes at once. So, focus on one area of change at a time. For instance, don't begin a new job, start a diet, and go on an exercise program all in the same week.

Try to divide large changes into small steps. For example, if you and your doctor decide you should begin a walking program of 45 minutes each day, don't expect to walk that long the first day. Begin by walking 10 or 15 minutes every other day. As you feel comfortable, gradually increase your walking to 20 minutes four or fives times a week. Don't worry if it takes several months for you to reach that 45-minutes-a-day goal.

By approaching changes gradually, you will increase your chance for success and diminish the opportunities for failure, frustration, and guilt.

Pat Yourself on the Back

We all are quick to criticize ourselves and feel guilty when we make a mistake. But many times we completely overlook our successes. For instance, you may not have worked on your exercise program for six months, but you have pretty much avoided inappropriate foods and kept to a healthy diet. So give yourself a pat on the back for sticking to the diet, rather than only knocking yourself for failing to do your exercises.

Even if it's not your tendency, you might benefit from taking stock of what you are doing well in relation to your diabetes. Sit down and make a list of everything you do every day just to control your diabetes. You might include

- I give myself injections or I take my pills.
- I monitor my blood glucose every day.
- I follow my meal plan.
- I exercise at least four times a week.
- I check my feet each evening.

The number of things you are already doing correctly and consistently—just to control diabetes—might surprise you. Give yourself credit for the effort you are making.

Making the effort to focus on your successes should help you feel better about yourself. And it's hard to feel guilty when you feel good about yourself. Keeping a daily journal of what you do right may even encourage you to take additional positive steps. You may develop a more objective appraisal of your diabetes management when you see it in black and white in your diary. Reviewing this record may help you counter discouragement and guilt when setbacks occur.

Failures Can Be Opportunities for Success

It may sound strange to look at a failure as an opportunity. Still, if you choose, you can use a failure as a chance to do better next time. A failure gives us an opportunity to reevaluate goals, to ask, "Is this a realistic goal for me right now?"

Failure also provides opportunities to think about alternative ways of approaching a problem. If what you are doing is not working, don't simply blame yourself. Try another approach.

Perhaps you and your doctor have decided that you should walk 15 minutes a day. You plan to take that walk at six each evening, but you realize after one walk that you are missing the one television show you really enjoy. Or, you might discover that the route you want to take has some loudly barking dogs that don't seem to be kept in the yard. Instead of watching the television show, not walking, and feeling guilty or telling yourself that you really can't face those dogs so you'd better not go out, make changes. See if you can take your walk right after the television show, then try walking in the opposite direction.

Give yourself credit for trying. Failure only comes to those who are trying to accomplish something in the first place.

It's possible to work for excellent diabetes self-care. It's impossible to be perfect all the time. Acknowledge that managing diabetes is not easy. Understand that you will not always be able to do everything you are supposed to do at the moment you should do it. You will make mistakes. But what counts is that you try your best as often as you can.

Appendix

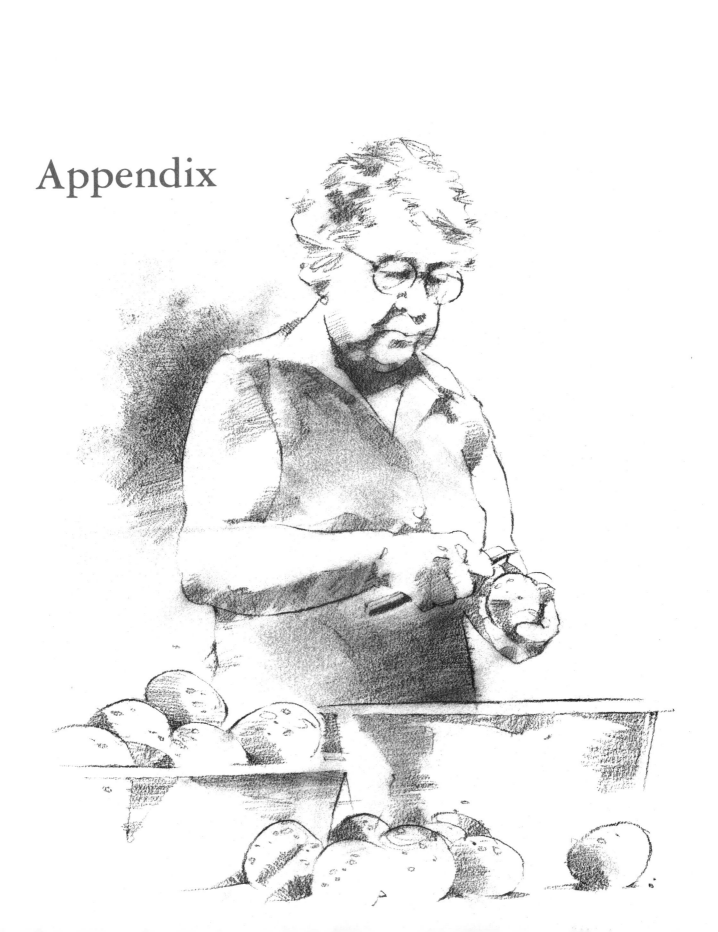

TO PERFORM SELF-MONITORING OF BLOOD GLUCOSE

Have ready a blood-letting device (lancet), a clean test strip, a cotton ball or tissue (if needed to wipe excess blood off test strip), a watch or other timing device, and a color chart for matching or a blood glucose meter. Make sure your hands are clean and dry.

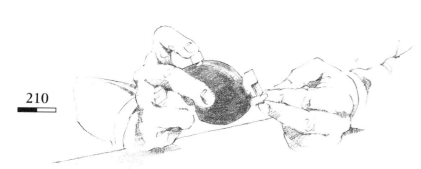

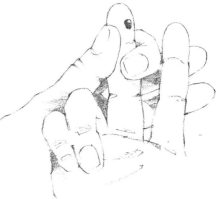

■ Puncture the skin of a finger with a lancet.

■ Squeeze out a large drop of blood.

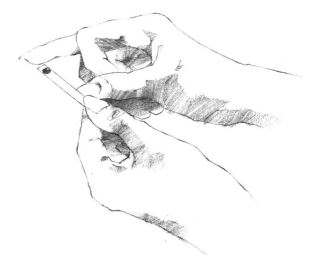

■ Place the blood drop on a test strip (or onto the sensor if your meter already has the test strip inside it). Wait the instructed amount of time for the test strip to develop.

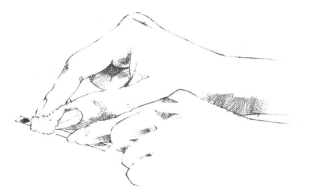

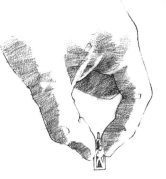

■ Wipe off excess blood, if instructed to do so, with a cotton ball or tissue. Then compare the test strip to the chart on the vial or insert the test strip into the meter. (With some meters, it is not necessary to wipe off the blood, and a smaller drop of blood will often do.)

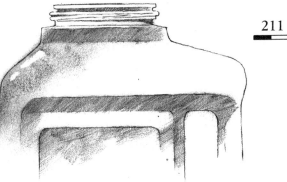

■ Dispose of the lancet with your syringe needles.

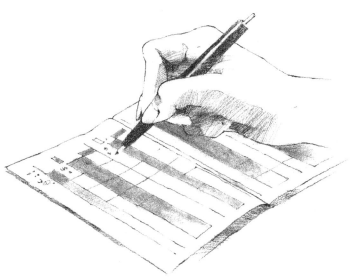

■ Be sure to record your finding.

To Prepare an Insulin Injection

To prepare your injection, you will need a sterile disposable syringe with needle, a bottle of insulin, clean hands and injection site, an alcohol swab (if desired to clean injection site or insulin bottle stopper), and something clean to set the filled syringe on while you prepare your injection site.

■ Make sure your hands are clean.

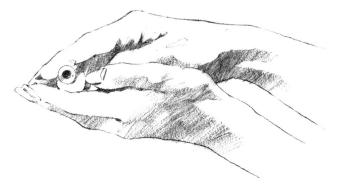

■ Roll any bottle of cloudy intermediate- or long-acting insulin between your hands. Don't shake it because this creates air bubbles in the insulin.

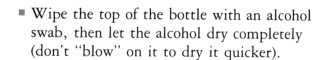

■ Wipe the top of the bottle with an alcohol swab, then let the alcohol dry completely (don't "blow" on it to dry it quicker).

■ Draw air into your syringe in an amount that matches your insulin dose.

■ Inject that amount of air into the insulin bottle.

■ Leaving the needle in the bottle, turn the bottle upside down so that the level of the insulin is above the end of the needle.

■ Pull the correct amount of insulin into the syringe.

■ Check for air bubbles on the inside of the syringe; if you see air bubbles, keep the bottle upside down and push the syringe plunger up so all the insulin is returned to the bottle.

■ Keep filling and emptying the syringe until the air bubbles are gone.

■ Remove the syringe from the bottle after checking again that you have the correct dose.

■ If you need to set the syringe down, place it on its side and make sure the needle doesn't touch anything.

TO PREPARE AN INSULIN MIXTURE

Your doctor may want you to inject two kinds of insulin at once using the same syringe. You would follow the methods given above with a couple of very important changes:

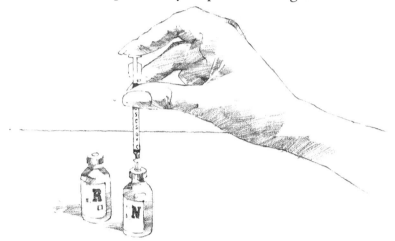

- First, inject air in the same amount as your dose (for instance, 30 units) into the intermediate- or long-acting insulin (the cloudy insulin)—do not remove any insulin. A word of caution: if you reuse your syringes, you want to prevent adding any short-acting insulin to your longer-acting insulin. You may want to inject a week's worth of air into your insulin vials when you are using a syringe for the first time.

- Next, inject air in the same amount as your dose (for instance, 10 units) into your short-acting insulin (the clear insulin), and keep the needle in this bottle.

■ Holding the bottle upside down, withdraw the correct amount of short-acting insulin.

■ Add the number of units of short-acting insulin to the number of units of longer-acting insulin you will with-draw next so you know the total units in your dose. For instance, 10 units short-acting insulin and 30 units intermediate-acting insulin equals 40 units total dose.

■ Insert your needle into the longer-acting insulin, holding the bottle upside down.

■ Withdraw the correct amount of insulin—remember to stop when you have withdrawn the calculated total dose of insulin. For instance, to add 30 units intermediate-acting insulin to the 10 units short-acting insulin already in the syringe, pull the plunger back to the 40-unit mark.

■ If you accidentally pull out too much of the second insulin, do not return it to the bottle—it will already be mixed. Discard the contents of your syringe and start again at the beginning.

If you are injecting insulin premixed by the manufacturer, such as a 70/30 mixture of intermediate- and short-acting insulin, roll the bottle gently between your hands before you fill your syringe to mix the insulins.

To Store Mixed Insulins

Some of the longer-acting (Lente and Ultralente) insulins contain a substance that causes the short-acting insulin to decrease its potency. For that reason, mixtures using these insulins must be injected immediately after mixing them to get the rapid action of Regular insulin.

You do not need to be concerned about changes in your insulin mixtures if you use NPH insulin. The potency of the Regular insulin is not affected by NPH insulin. You can inject the mixed insulins right away or store the mixture in the syringe in the refrigerator. Mixtures stored in the syringe must be gently rolled between the hands before they are injected. This remixes the two kinds of insulin.

This guideline also does not apply to insulin that comes premixed from the manufacturer. These mixtures will be stable, although the bottle they come in should be rolled between the hands before drawing out the dose.

To Inject Insulin

You will need a filled sterile syringe, a clean injection site, and a sterile cotton ball or gauze square, if desired, to cover the injection site for a few seconds after the injection. Insulin is injected into fatty tissue and then absorbed into surrounding muscles. See Chapter 3 for insulin injection sites.

■ Gently pinch a fold of skin between your thumb and forefinger and inject straight in.

216

■ Push the needle through the skin as quickly as you can.

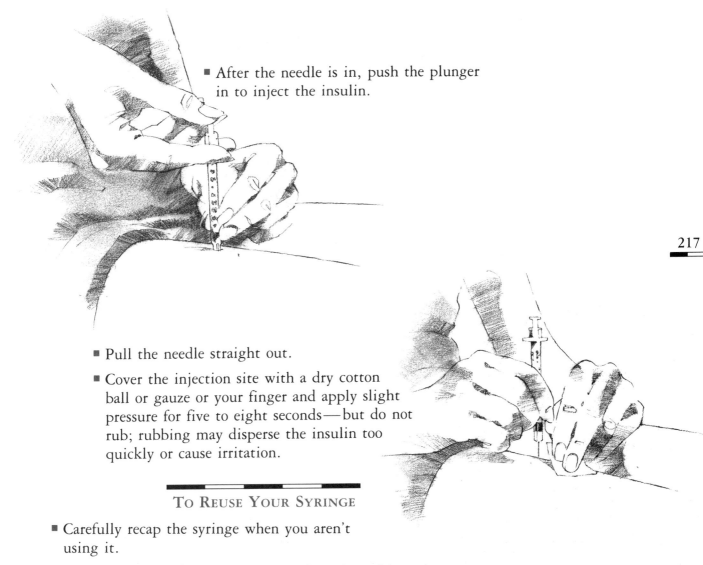

■ After the needle is in, push the plunger in to inject the insulin.

■ Pull the needle straight out.

■ Cover the injection site with a dry cotton ball or gauze or your finger and apply slight pressure for five to eight seconds—but do not rub; rubbing may disperse the insulin too quickly or cause irritation.

To Reuse Your Syringe

■ Carefully recap the syringe when you aren't using it.

■ Don't let the needle touch anything but clean skin and your insulin bottle stopper. If it touches anything else, don't reuse it.

■ Store the used syringe at room temperature.

■ There will always be a tiny, even invisible, amount of insulin left in the syringe—so use particular syringes with just one type of insulin to avoid mixing insulins.

- Do not reuse a needle that is bent or dull. However, just because an injection is painful doesn't mean the needle is dull—you may have hit a nerve ending or have wet alcohol on your skin, if you use alcohol to clean the injection site.

- Do not wipe your needle with alcohol—this may remove the coating that makes for less painful injections.

- When you're finished with a syringe, dispose of it responsibly. See the guidelines in Chapter 3.

Resources for People With Type II Diabetes

PUBLICATIONS ON MEAL PLANNING

From the American Diabetes Association:

For information on how to order these publications, call the ADA at (800) 232-3472, ext. 363.

Month of Meals Twenty-eight days of breakfasts, lunches, and dinners that figure your calories and exchanges for you. There are step-by-step instructions for adapting the meals to calorie levels that match your needs. Also included is a selection of delicious snacks. Many menus include easy, healthy recipes. A special section gives menus for special occasions.

Month of Meals 2 Another 28 days of healthy, delicious meals already planned for you. This edition gives quick-to-fix and ethnic meals and has a special section on making healthy food choices that meet your meal plan when you are dining out at Mexican, Italian, Chinese, and fast food restaurants.

Month of Meals 3 More healthy meals, featuring high-fiber and convenience foods that fit into your busy lifestyle and menus for when you need a quick meal away from home. Information on smart grocery store shopping, wise fast food choices, and healthy menus for picnics and barbecues fills the pages.

Exchange Lists for Meal Planning Colorful charts, helpful tips on good nutrition, and an introduction to the six easy-to-use food Exchange Lists show you how to balance your diet and gain control over diabetes. (Also available in large print.)

Eating Healthy Foods This booklet provides an introduction to making daily food choices for breakfast, lunch, dinner, and snacks using the Exchange Lists.

Family Cookbook, Volume I More than 250 delicious, economical, kitchen-tested recipes fill these cookbook. It offers an encyclopedia of nutrition information, tips on eating out, brown-bagging, weight control, exercise, and more.

Family Cookbook, Volume II This volume includes ways to cut sugar, calories, and costs—plus there are more than 250 tasty recipes. It has an entire section devoted to living with diabetes and gives advice on the emotional aspects of dieting.

Family Cookbook, Volume III Two hundred more recipes to add to your eating pleasure. This cookbook gives tips on microwaving, food processing, and freezing for fix-ahead meals. Also included are recipes for eating ethnic cuisines.

Family Cookbook, Volume IV, The American Tradition Recipes from Boston Scrod to Santa Fe Chicken (more than 200 recipes in all) fill each page of this new cookbook with great American flavor. There is a colorful introductory section of interesting facts about the history of American cuisine.

American Diabetes Association Holiday Cookbook and *American Diabetes Association Special Celebrations and Parties Cookbook*, both by Betty Wedman, MS, RD Start a family tradition of healthier eating for all your special occasions. These books provide you with recipes for delicious and nutritious foods that your entire family will enjoy.

Meal Planning With Jewish Foods and *Meal Planning With Mexican-American Foods* (also available in Spanish) These pamphlets provide practical tips for including traditional ethnic foods in your diabetes meal plan.

From Other Publishers:

Fast Food Facts by Marion J. Franz, RD, MS (DCI/CHRONIMED Publishing, PO Box 47945, Minneapolis, MN 55447; 1990) Nutritive and Exchange values for fast food restaurants.

Convenience Food Facts by Arlene Monk, RD, CDE, and Marion J. Franz, RD, MS (DCI/CHRONIMED Publishing, PO Box 47945, Minneapolis, MN 55447; 1991) Nutritive and Exchange values for grocery store items by brand name.

Exchanges for All Occasions by Marion J. Franz, RD, MS (DCI/CHRONIMED Publishing, PO Box 47945, Minneapolis, MN 55447; 1987) Nutritive and Exchange values for everyday foods.

The Restaurant Companion by Hope S. Warshaw, MMSc, RD (Surrey Books, 101 East Erie Street, Suite 900, Chicago, IL 60611; 1990) A guide to eating out the healthy way.

Eat for Life: The Food and Nutrition Board's Guide to Reducing Your Risk of Chronic Disease Catherine E. Woteki, PhD, RD, and Paul R. Thomas, EdD, RD (Editors) (National Academy Press, 2101 Constitution Avenue, NW, PO Box 285, Washington, DC 20055; 1992) Easy-to-understand version of National Academy of Sciences nutrition guidelines for good health.

Other Sources for Food-Related Information:

For information on proper food handling:
U.S. Department of Agriculture
(800) 535-4555 weekdays 10–4 EST

To obtain the pamphlet *How to Read a Label* (HHS publication number 80-1065), write to:
U.S. Department of Health and Human Services
Public Health Service, Food and Drug Administration
Rockville, MD 20857

PUBLICATIONS FOR BETTER LIVING WITH DIABETES

From the American Diabetes Association:

For information on how to order these publications, call the ADA at (800) 232-3472, ext. 363.

Diabetes: A to Z This dictionary-style book answers your questions about lifestyle, nutrition, exercise, and much more in clear, easy-to-understand terms.

The 'Other' Diabetes This lively and colorful book provides practical advice and inspiration as you follow one man's experience with type II diabetes.

Buyer's Guide to Diabetes Products Updated every year to reflect new products and diabetes care breakthroughs, this guide compares features from different manufacturers for everything from insulin, syringes, and jet injectors to insulin pumps and test strips. Available as a reprint from *Diabetes Forecast*.

The Journey and the Dream: A History of the American Diabetes Association Written for ADA's 50th anniversary, this book tells the intertwining story of progress in caring for people with diabetes and the mission of the ADA.

From Another Publisher:

Diabetes, Visual Impairment, and Group Support: A Guidebook by Judith Caditz, PhD (The Center for the Partially Sighted, 720 Wilshire Boulevard, Suite 200, Santa Monica, CA 90401-1713; 1988) Information on how to deal with both the physical and emotional problems of visual impairment.

SERVICE AND SUPPORT GROUPS

Membership in the American Diabetes Association

ADA's members-only magazine, *Diabetes Forecast*, helps you better understand and control your diabetes, so you enjoy more of the good things in life. Each month, *Diabetes Forecast* is filled with updates on advances in diabetes research, treatment, and easier self-care, advice on coping with daily stress, information on safe ways to exercise, and delicious easy-to-fix recipes. Introduce yourself to others who share your concerns and also live with the challenge of diabetes.

Diabetes Forecast in one of the many benefits of ADA membership. To receive more information on membership in the ADA, call (800) 232-3472, ext. 343, for membership services.

Although your best resource for information is likely to be your local ADA Affiliate listed in the white pages of your telephone book, the resources listed below may offer important additional services and/or information.

For the Visually Challenged:

American Council of the Blind
1155 15th Street, NW
Suite 720
Washington, DC 20005
(202) 467-5081
(800) 424-8666
National information clearinghouse and legislative advocate that publishes a bimonthly newsletter in Braille, large print, and cassette versions.

American Foundation for the Blind
15 West 16th Street
New York, NY 10011
(212) 620-2000
(800) 232-5463
Works to establish, develop, and provide services and programs that assist visually challenged people in achieving independence.

American Printing House for the Blind
1839 Frankfort Avenue
PO Box 6085
Louisville, KY 40206
(502) 895-2405
Concerned with the publication of literature in all media (Braille, large type, recorded) and manufacture of educational aids. Newsletter provides information on new products.

Bible Alliance, Inc.
PO Box 621
Bradenton, FL 34206
(813) 748-3031
Cassette albums of scripture in 38 languages.

Blinded Veterans Association
477 H Street, NW
Washington, DC 20001
(202) 371-8880
Assists veterans blinded during military service in attaining employment and reestablishing themselves in their communities.

Division for the Blind and Visually Impaired
Rehabilitation Service Administration
Department of Education
Room 3229
Mary Switzer Building
330 C Street, SW
Washington, DC 20202
(202) 732-1316
Provides rehabilitative training, through agencies in each state, to those who have become visually impaired who wish to maintain their employment or train for new employment.

Carroll Center for the Blind
770 Centre Street
Newton, MA 02158
(617) 969-6200
Rehabilitation training, counseling, outdoor enrichment program, work evaluation, and diagnostic assessments.

G.K. Hall and Company
Large Print Books
70 Lincoln Street
Boston, MA 02111
(617) 423-3990
(800) 343-2806
Free catalog of books in large print.

Illinois Society for the Prevention of Blindness
407 S. Dearborn
Suite 1000
Chicago, IL 60605
(312) 922-8710
Information for sighted people at risk for blindness.

National Association for Visually Handicapped (NAVH)
22 West 21st Street
New York, NY 10010
(212) 889-3141
or
NAVH San Francisco regional office
3201 Balboa Street
San Francisco, CA 94121
(415) 221-3201
List of low-vision facilities available by state. Visual aid counseling and visual aids, peer support groups, and more intensive counseling offered at regional offices. Some counseling done by mail or phone.

National Braille Press
88 St. Stephen Street
Boston, MA 02115
(617) 266-6160 (voice)
(617) 437-0456 (fax)
(800) 548-7323
Catalog available.

National Federation of the Blind
1800 Johnson Street
Baltimore, MD 21230
(410) 659-9314
(800) 638-7518 (toll-free number only for job opportunities for the blind)
Service resources offered through state chapters of this membership

223

organization. Some aids and appliances available through national headquarters. The Diabetics Division publishes a quarterly newsletter.

National Library Service (NLS) for the Physically Handicapped
Library of Congress
1291 Taylor Street, NW
Washington, DC 20542
(202) 707-5100
(800) 424-8567 (to speak with a reference person)
(800) 424-9100 (to leave a message)
Bimonthly magazine *Encore*, which includes articles from *Diabetes Forecast*, available on request through the NLS program to regional and state libraries.

Recordings for the Blind (RFB)
20 Roszel Road
Princeton, NJ 08540
(609) 452-0606 (voice)
(609) 987-8116 (fax)
(800) 221-4792 (weekdays 9–9 EST)
Audiotape library for print-handicapped registered with RFB. Free loan of cassettes for up to a year. 80,000 titles on cassette.

Seeing Eye Guide Dogs
PO Box 375
Morristown, NJ 07963-0375
(201) 539-4425 (voice)
(201) 993-1714 (fax)
Guide dog training and instruction on working with a guide dog.

Vision Foundation, Inc.
818 Mount Auburn Street
Watertown, MA 02172
(617) 926-4232
National resource list. Self-help program in local area and buddy system throughout the state of Massachusetts.

Vision Services for the Blind
817 Broadway
New York, NY 10003
Rehabilitation program that teaches independent living skills for New York City area residents.

For Amputees:

American Amputee Foundation
PO Box 250218
Little Rock, AR 72225
(501) 666-2523
Peer counseling to new amputees and their families. Information and referral.

National Amputation Foundation
12-45 150th Street
Whitestone, NY 11357
(718) 767-0596 (voice)
(718) 767-3103 (fax)
Sponsor of Amp-to-Amp program in which new amputee is visited by amputee who has resumed normal life. List of support groups throughout the country available.

For Those Needing Long-Term or Home Care:

Nursing Home Information Service
c/o National Council of Senior Citizens
925 15th Street, NW
Washington, DC 20005
(202) 347-8800
Information on selecting and paying for a nursing home.

National Association for Home Care
519 C Street, NE
Washington, DC 20002
(202) 547-7424
Information on and advocacy promoting high standards of home health care.

224

OTHER HEALTH-RELATED INFORMATION SOURCES OR SERVICES

Sources for Finding Quality Health Care:

American Medical Association
515 North State Street
Chicago 60610
(312) 464-4818
Will tell you how to contact your county or state medical society, which will provide you with a referral to a local physician.

American Board of Medical
  Specialties
1 Rotary Center, Suite 805
Evanston, IL 60201
(708) 491-9091
(800) 776-2378
Record of physicians certified by 24 medical specialty boards. Certification status of physician available to callers. Directories of certified physicians organized by city of medical practice and alphabetically by physician names available in many libraries.

American Association for Marriage
  and Family Therapy
1100 17th Street, NW, 10th Floor
Washington, DC 20036
(202) 452-0109
(800) 374-2638
Referral to local professional marriage and family therapist.

National Association of Social
  Workers
750 First Street, NE
Suite 700
Washington, DC 20002
(202) 408-8600
(800) 638-8799
Referral to local professional social worker.

American Association of Diabetes
  Educators
444 North Michigan Avenue, Suite
  1240
Chicago, IL 60611
(312) 644-2233
(800) 338-3633
Referral to local professional diabetes educator.

The American Dietetic Association
216 West Jackson Boulevard, Suite
  800
Chicago, IL 60606
(312) 899-0040
(800) 877-1600
Information, guidance, and referral to local professional dietitians.

American Optometric Association
243 N. Lindbergh Boulevard
St. Louis, MO 63141
(314) 991-4100
Referral to state optometric association for local referral to professional optometrist.

National Eye Care Program
(800) 222-3937
Assists U.S. citizens over age 65 who do not have access to an ophthalmologist and cannot afford care.

American Board of Podiatric
  Surgery
1601 Dolores Street
San Francisco, CA 94110
(415) 826-3200
Referral to board-certified local podiatrist.

For Miscellaneous Health Information:

24-Hour Counseling Line (suicide, depression):
Humanistic Foundation
(800) 999-4572

National AIDS Hotline:
(800) 458-5231
(800) 344-7432 (Spanish)

For referral to local affiliate's Heartline, which provides information on cardiovascular health and disease prevention:
American Heart Association
(800) 242-8721

For brochures on eye care and eye diseases, send a self-addressed, stamped envelope to:
American Academy of
  Ophthalmology
Customer Service Department
PO Box 7424
San Francisco, CA 94120-7424
(415) 561-8500

To order *Health Information for International Travelers*:
Centers for Disease Control, U.S. Government Printing Office, stock no. 017-023-00189-2
(202) 783-3238

For a list of doctors in foreign countries who speak English and who received postgraduate training in North America or Great Britain:
International Association for Medical Assistance to Travelers
350 5th Avenue, Suite 5620
New York, NY 10001
(716) 754-4883

For a list of International Diabetes Federation groups that can offer assistance when you're traveling:
International Diabetes Federation
40 Washington Street
B-1050 Brussels, Belgium

For information, guidance, and physician referral in each state on impotence:
Impotence Institute of America
(800) 669-1603

For a free copy of *One Step at a Time*, an information guide on running:
President's Council on Physical Fitness
(202) 272-3430

To learn more about chronic pain and how to deal with it:
National Chronic Pain Outreach Association
(301) 652-4948

For People Over 50:

American Association for Retired Persons (AARP)
601 E Street, NW
Washington, DC 20049
(202) 434-2277
Pharmacy (800) 456-2277
Prescriptions mailed to your door. Prices the same for members and nonmembers. $1 postage and shipping per order. Possible savings over drugstore prices on generic drugs, but no prices are guaranteed.

National Council on the Aging
409 3rd Street, 2nd Floor
Washington, DC 20024
(202) 479-1200
Advocacy group concerned with developing and implementing high standards of care for the elderly. Referral to local agencies concerned with the elderly.

Sources for Health Insurance Information

Medicare Hotline
(800) 638-6833

The Medicare Handbook is available from:
Medicare Publications
Health Care Financing Administration
6325 Security Boulevard
Baltimore, MD 21207

Free Medicare/Medicaid counseling referral services from the AARP:
(202) 434-2241

Health insurance through the AARP:
(800) 523-5800
Individuals with diabetes or other chronic illnesses are eligible for health insurance if applicant is within 6 months of 65th birthday. A 3-month waiting period is required for those with conditions preexistent in the 6 months preceding the effective date of the insurance.

State Insurance Commissions or Departments

Some states have formed insurance risk pools to make it possible for individuals to obtain health insurance regardless of their state of health. In the list below, states are divided according to whether they do or do not have risk-pooled insurance. If your state is not listed as having risk-pooled insurance, check with your state's insurance department. Some states may have adopted such an insurance program since August 1, 1992.

In states preceded with a single asterisk, inquiries should be directed to Commissioner of Insurance, Department of Insurance. In states preceded with a double asterisk, inquiries should be directed to Director of Insurance, Department of Insurance. For states where job title and department name varies from these, the correct forms are included with the address.

States With Insurance Risk Pools as of August 1, 1991:

*California
100 Van Ness Avenue
San Francisco, CA 94102
(415) 557-1126

*Colorado
303 West Colfax Avenue, Suite 500
Denver, CO 80204
(303) 620-4300

*Connecticut
165 Capitol Avenue, PO Box 816
Hartford, CT 06142-0816
(203) 297-3800

Florida
Commissioner of Insurance and Treasurer
Department of Insurance
Larson Building
Tallahassee, FL 32301
(904) 488-3440

*Georgia
7th Floor, West Tower
No. 2 Martin Luther King Jr. Drive
Atlanta, GA 30334
(404) 656-2056

**Illinois
320 West Washington Street
Springfield, IL 62767
(217) 782-4515

*Indiana
311 West Washington, Suite 300
Indianapolis, IN 46204-2787
(317) 232-2385

*Iowa
Lucas State Office Building
Des Moines, IA 50319
(515) 281-5705

*Louisiana
PO Box 44214, Capitol Station
Baton Rouge, LA 70804
(504) 342-5322

Maine
Superintendent of Insurance
Bureau of Insurance
State House Station 34
Augusta, ME 04333
(207) 582-8707

Minnesota
Commissioner of Commerce
Department of Commerce
133 E. 7th Street
St. Paul, MN 55101
(612) 296-4026

*Mississippi
PO Box 79
Jackson, MS 39205
(601) 359-3569

**Missouri
PO Box 690
Jefferson City, MO 65102
(314) 751-4126

Montana
State Auditor and Commissioner of Insurance
Department of Insurance
Mitchell Building, PO Box 4009
Helena, MT 59604-4009
(406) 444-2040

**Nebraska
Terminal Building
941 O Street, Suite 400
Lincoln, NE 68508
(402) 471-2201

New Mexico
Superintendent of Insurance
Department of Insurance
PO Box 1269
Sante Fe, NM 87504-1269
(505) 827-4500

*North Dakota
600 East Boulevard
Bismarck, ND 58505-0158
(701) 224-2440

*Oregon
21 Labor & Industries Building
Salem, OR 97310
(503) 378-4271

Rhode Island
Commissioner of Insurance
Department of Business Regulation
233 Richmond Street, Suite 233
Providence, RI 02903-4233
(401) 277-2223

*South Carolina
PO Box 100105
1612 Marion Street
Columbia, SC 29202-3105
(803) 737-6160

*Tennessee
500 James Robertson Parkway
Nashville, TN 37243-0560
(615) 741-2241

Texas
Commissioner of Insurance
State Board of Insurance
PO Box 149104
Austin, TX 78714-9104
(512) 463-6169

*Utah
3110 State Office Building
Salt Lake City, UT 84145
(801) 538-3800

*Washington
Insurance Building AQ-21
Olympia, WA 98504-0321
(206) 753-7300

*Wisconsin
PO Box 7873
121 E. Wilson
Madison, WI 53707-7873
(608) 266-3585

*Wyoming
Herschler Building
122 West 25th Street
Cheyenne, WY 82002-0440
(307) 777-7401

States Without Insurance Risk Pools as of August 1, 1991:

*Alabama
135 South Union Street
Montgomery, AL 36130-3401
(205) 269-3550

Alaska
Director of Insurance
Department of Commerce
Division of Insurance, Pouch "D"
Juneau, AK 99811
(907) 465-2515

**Arizona
3030 N. 3rd Street, Suite 1100
Phoenix, AZ 85012
(602) 255-5400

*Arkansas
400 University Tower Building
Little Rock, AR 72204
(501) 686-2900

*Delaware
841 Silver Lake Boulevard
Dover, DE 19901
(302) 736-4251

District of Columbia
Superintendent of Insurance
Department of Insurance
613 G Street, 6th Floor
Washington, DC 20001
(202) 727-8000

Hawaii
Commissioner of Insurance
Hawaii Division of Insurance
Department of Commerce &
    Consumer Affairs
PO Box 3614
Honolulu, HI 96811
(808) 586-2790

**Idaho
500 South 10th Street
Boise, ID 83720
(208) 334-2250

*Kansas
420 S.W. 9th Street
Topeka, KS 66612
(913) 296-3071

*Kentucky
PO Box 517, 229 West Main
    Street
Frankfort, KY 40602
(502) 564-3630

Maryland
Commissioner of Insurance
Department of Licensing and
    Regulation
501 St. Paul Place
Baltimore, MD 21202-2272
(301) 659-4027

*Massachusetts
280 Friend Street
Boston, MA 02114
(617) 727-7189

228

Michigan
Commissioner of Insurance
Department of Licensing and
   Regulation
PO Box 30220
Ottawa Building North, 2nd Floor
Lansing, MI 48909
(517) 373-0220

*Nevada
1665 Hot Springs Road
Carson City, NV 89710
(702) 486-4009

*New Hampshire
GAA Plaza, 169 Manchester Street
Concord, NH 03301
(603) 271-2261 through 2267

*New Jersey
20 West State Street, CN-325
Trenton, NJ 08625-0325
(609) 292-5363

New York
Superintendent of Insurance
Department of Insurance
106 West Broadway
New York, NY 10013
(212) 602-0428

*North Carolina
PO Box 26387, Dobbs Building
430 N. Salisbury Street
Raleigh, NC 27611
(919) 733-7343

**Ohio
2100 Stella Court
Columbus, OH 43266-0566
(614) 644-2658

*Oklahoma
PO Box 53408
Oklahoma City, OK 73105
(405) 521-2828

*Pennsylvania
1326 Strawberry Square
Harrisburg, PA 17120
(717) 787-5173

*Puerto Rico
PO Box 8330
Fernandez Juncos Station
Santurce, PR 00910
(809) 722-8686

**South Dakota
Commerce Building
910 E. Sioux Avenue
Pierce, SD 57501
(605) 773-3563

Vermont
Commissioner of Insurance
Department of Banking, Insurance,
   and Securities
City Center Building, 89 Main
   Street
Montpelier, VT 05602-3101
(802) 828-3301

Virginia
Commissioner of Insurance
Bureau of Insurance
State Corporation Commission
PO Box 1157
Richmond, VA 23209
(804) 786-3741

*West Virginia
Commissioner of Insurance
Department of Insurance
2019 Washington Street East
Charleston, WV 25305
(304) 348-3394

229

OTHER USEFUL INFORMATION SOURCES OR SERVICES

Social Security Administration
(800) 772-1213

For help with taxes for the elderly,
those with a disability, those
for whom English is a second
language:
Internal Revenue Service
(800) 829-1040

For a catalog of clothing designed
for people in wheelchairs or with
limited mobility:
Avenues
(800) 848-2837 or from Canada
   call collect to (805) 388-7668

To order a medical ID
bracelet:
Medic Alert Foundation
PO Box 1009
Turlock, CA 95381-1009
(800) 432-5378

Index